Ankylosing Spondylitis - Recent Concepts

Edited by Jácome Bruges Armas

Published in London, United Kingdom

Ankylosing Spondylitis - Recent Concepts
http://dx.doi.org/10.5772/intechopen.98070
Edited by Jácome Bruges Armas

Contributors
Razvan Adrian Ionescu, Horatiu Popoviciu, Florentin Ananu Vreju, Esra Dilsat Bayrak, Malini Alexander, Rajeshwar Nath Srivastava, Shatakshi Pant, Sudeepti Ratan Srivastava, Amar Chandra Sharma, Saloni Raj, Jácome Bruges Armas

First published in London, United Kingdom, 2023 by IntechOpen
IntechOpen is the global imprint of INTECHOPEN LIMITED, registered in England and Wales, registration number: 11086078, 5 Princes Gate Court, London, SW7 2QJ, United Kingdom

British Library Cataloguing-in-Publication Data
A catalogue record for this book is available from the British Library

Additional hard and PDF copies can be obtained from orders@intechopen.com

Ankylosing Spondylitis - Recent Concepts
Edited by Jácome Bruges Armas
p. cm.
Print ISBN 978-1-80356-242-1
Online ISBN 978-1-80356-243-8
eBook (PDF) ISBN 978-1-80356-244-5

Meet the editor

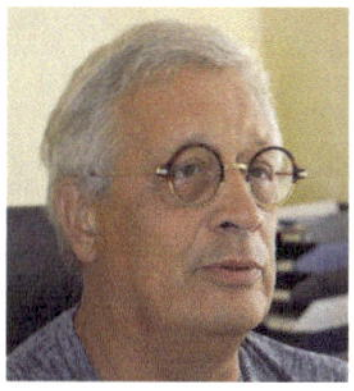

Dr. Jácome Bruges Armas is a senior specialist in internal medicine and a board-certified medical specialist in medical oncology by the Portuguese Medical Council. He is currently the director of the Epidemiology and Molecular Biology Service (SEEBMO) at the Hospital de Santo Espirito de Angra do Heroísmo, Terceira Island, Azores, Portugal. He is also a researcher at the Comprehensive Health Research Centre (CHRC), Lisbon, Portugal. His research interests include the epidemiology and molecular genetics of spondylarthritis (SpA), diffuse idiopathic skeletal hyperostosis (DISH), and chondrocalcinosis (CC). He is a member of several scientific organizations and a member of the editorial board of several scientific journals. He has published more than 100 peer-reviewed publications, including journal articles, conference papers, books, and book chapters.

Contents

Preface

Research in the last decades has provided new data improving the knowledge of the clinical findings, pathogenesis, and treatment of ankylosing spondylitis (AS). Magnetic resonance imaging (MRI) has helped to define two subsets of axial spondylarthritis (ax SpA) that may be considered different presentations of the same disease: non-radiographic ax SpA, which does not fulfill the radiographic criteria of the modified New York criteria, and radiographic ax SpA, which does fulfill the radiographic criteria of the modified New York criteria. Another important finding was reported in 2010, which showed that although most patients with AS have elevated levels of the inflammatory markers erythrocyte sedimentation rate (ESR) and C-reactive protein (CRP), some patients may have active disease with normal levels of these markers. These findings are clearly important for treatment decisions.

This book presents updated data on the diagnosis, pathogenesis, and treatment of AS. Section 1, "History, Classification Criteria and Imaging in AS", includes three chapters that describe how AS patients are characterized using metrology, functional indexes, diagnostic criteria, and imaging.

Chapter 1, "Introductory Chapter: AS Times Go by – An Axial Chronicle", is dedicated to the history of the first descriptions of AS by Bernard Connor, followed by those of Strumpell, Von Bechterew, and Pierre Marie. The chapter chronicles the evolution of the diagnostic criteria over time, starting with the Rome criteria in 1961, which used objective clinical methods to measure spinal mobility. The New York criteria introduced sacroiliitis, which is considered the hallmark of AS. These criteria were modified by van der Linden in 1984, expanding the diagnostic criteria to non-axial spondyloarthropathies. The Amor and the European Spondylarthritis Study Group (ESSG) criteria were developed in 1990, followed by the Assessment of Spondylarthritis International Society (ASAS) criteria, which defined the two subsets of ax SpA.

This chapter also examines metrology and self-administered questionnaires, including the test by Schoeber (1937), the Health Assessment Questionnaire (HAQ score), and the Bath indexes (BASDAI, BASFI, and BASMI) developed by Andrei Calin et al. at the Royal National Hospital for Rheumatic Diseases, Bath, UK, all of which are important contributions to AS characterization and research. The chapter also examines the mechanisms involved in AS pathogenesis, including major histocompatibility complex (MHC) alleles, non-MHC genetic associations, and new treatments targeting some of these genes.

Chapter 2, "Diagnostic/Classification Criteria", deals with the diagnostic and classification criteria of AS, emphasizing that they have different goals. While diagnostic criteria should be used to diagnose AS, classification criteria are intended to be used in already diagnosed patients, mainly for research purposes. As we know, the modified diagnostic criteria may fail to detect early AS, and MRI that helps to visualize early bone marrow oedema led to the development of the ASAS classification criteria. According to the authors, the ASAS criteria have a specificity of 84.4% and a sensitivity of 82.9% and represent a major step forward for ax SpA. In clinical practice, most rheumatologists use the ASAS criteria for diagnostic purposes because it may ease the diagnostic process since they represent the most frequently encountered characteristics of the disease. Overdiagnosis may be a negative consequence of using classification criteria for diagnostic purposes.

Chapter 3, "Imaging Ankylosing Spondylitis", discusses imaging in AS. Conventional radiography remains an important tool for the diagnosis of structural changes in the sacroiliac joints (SIJs) and spine. According to the New York criteria, the SIJs findings have a high specificity but low sensitivity for ax SpA, especially in early disease. Syndesmophytes and ankylosis of the spine are almost pathognomonic of AS, and syndesmophytes are the best predictors of radiographic progression. Scoring systems include the Modified Stoke Ankylosing Spondylitis Spinal Score (mSASSS) and the Bath Ankylosing Spondylitis Radiology Index (BASRI). The first is derived from the sum of scores for the lumbar and cervical spine. The second may be subdivided into BASRI-s for the spine only, BASRI-h for the hips, and BASRI-T for the summation of both. For the lumbar spine is a composite of lateral and anteroposterior views, for the cervical spine only the spine lateral view is scored. mSASSS is the preferred scoring method to evaluate the radiographic progression of AS.

Computed tomography (CT) shows chronic changes more clearly than conventional radiography and permits imaging of structural changes without superposition of overlying structures. The main value of CT is to document erosions of bone at any joint or enthesis and documenting fractures, but unlike MRI it does not reveal bone marrow oedema.

MRI can detect both active inflammatory and structural changes like bone marrow oedema and osteitis and is particularly useful for the early diagnosis of AS and for classifying patients with SpA. The SPARCC method is the most used to score the MRI and is based on the evaluation of the stir sequences of six consecutive semicoronal slices focusing on the synovial part of the SIJ.

Ultrasonography is a noninvasive, low-cost, and highly operator-dependent technique that is very useful in the diagnosis of peripheral involvement of the disease. It is also used as a guide for intra-articular treatment in peripheral joints as well as SIJs. Bone scintigraphy has a limited value in clinical practice, but quality and specificity may be increased using single-photon emission CT (SPECT).

Section 2, "Pathogenesis and Treatment of Ankylosing Spondylitis", includes two chapters that update our knowledge about the role of genetics, immunological factors, and infections and the enteric microbiome on AS pathogenesis.

Chapter 4, "Ankylosing Spondylitis Pathogenesis and Pathophysiology", examines the role of genetic factors in AS. HLA-B27 has 223 subtypes and is the most common recognizable susceptibility genetic factor for AS; however, it accounts for only around 20% of AS development, suggesting that other factors are also responsible. Other HLA genes have been recognized as being AS-associated, and many other non-HLA genes have been identified, namely, ERAP1, ERAP2, NPEPPS, IL23R, and KIRLR genes. Genetic variants and expression levels of TLR4 implicate innate immunity in the pathogenesis of AS and support the concept that AS has autoinflammatory components in its physiopathology. Immune pathways such as autophagy and ubiquitination and inflammasome are involved in both innate and adaptative response, and innate and innate-like immune cells can be found at sites of disease, likely representing the major source of IL-17 production in AS. Both autoimmune (the production of specific autoantibodies is very well-known in AS) and autoinflammatory factors are probably involved in AS pathogenesis.

Finally, Chapter 5, "Treatment Modalities of Ankylosing Spondylitis", discusses the treatment modalities for controlling AS. It describes the treatment of AS across the years, focusing on the use of biologic drugs that block inflammatory cytokines, halt disease progression, and improve patient quality of life. The chapter first discusses nonpharmacological treatment, including individual home-based or supervised exercise programs, including Yoga, which are internationally accepted as a good strategy for AS treatment. The chapter next discusses pharmacological treatments, including nonsteroidal anti-inflammatory drugs (NSAIDs) and different types of disease-modifying antirheumatic drugs (DMARDs) as second-line treatment for patients with AS. A substantial part of the chapter is dedicated to cytokine therapy, which is classified into three groups: TNF inhibitors (infliximab, etanercept, adalimumab, golimumab, and certolizumab), IL inhibitors (secukinumab and ixekizumab,) and JAK1 and 3 inhibitors (tofacitinib and upadacitinib) A last point is dedicated to therapies under study, including ustekinumab, a humanized IgG1k mAB that binds to p40-subunit shared by IL-12 and IL23, and stem cell therapy.

Jácome Bruges Armas MD, Ph.D.
Epidemiology and Molecular Biology Service (SEEBMO),
Hospital de Santo Espirito de Angra do Heroísmo,
Terceira Island, The Azores, Portugal

Comprehensive Health Research Centre (CHRC),
Nova Medical School,
University of Lisbon,
Lisbon, Portugal

Section 1

History, Classification Criteria and Imaging in AS

Chapter 1

Introductory Chapter: AS Times Go by – An Axial Chronicle

Jácome Bruges Armas

1. Introduction

The first description of Ankylosing Spondylitis (AS) is assigned to Bernard Connor, a Medical Doctor, born in Ireland in 1666, who attended the Medical Schools of Paris, Montpellier and Reims. He found a skeleton in a graveyard in which the ilium and sacrum and the 15 lowest vertebral and adjoining ribs formed one continuous bone. This finding was reported in three different languages—French, Latin and English (1691–1695).

The classical description of AS was published by Strumpell (1884) describing two patients with complete ankylosis of the spine and hip joints [1]. This first description was followed by another paper of Strumpell (1897) [2], two papers of von Bechterew (1893 and 1899) [3, 4] and one paper of Pierre Marie (1898) [5]. This last author is agreed to have given the most detailed clinical description together with his pupil, Léri, which gave a detailed pathological description based on two autopsies (1899 and 1926) [6, 7].

During the next years, after Roentgen developed X-rays (1895), many descriptions were written in different languages and countries together with radiological descriptions of the spine. Surprisingly, sacroiliac disease, a hallmark of AS, was not fully recognised until 1930 [8–11].

After the First and Second World Wars, new data were recognised, resulting from the screening and pensionability of young adults. It was found that women were also affected, and that AS was a familial disease, sometimes involving psoriasis, Reiter's disease [12], iritis, ulcerative colitis and Crohn's disease, heart and lung complications, and neurological complications, namely, long tract lesions due to atlanto-occipital and atlanto-axial subluxations and to a cauda equina syndrome associated with arachnoiditis. To investigate AS as a familial disease, with ethnic differences, new tissue antigenic techniques were applied (human leucocyte antigen (HLA) system), and a major breakthrough resulted with a strong association between AS and the allele HLA-B27, published independently in 1973 by Schlosstein et al. [13] and Brewerton et al. [14]. The development of the population survey techniques firmly established familial aggregation [15] and racial differences [16].

During the last years, some modifications in the terminology have been introduced. AS (axial spondyloarthritis (axSpA)) is now included in the Spondyloarthritis (SpA), a group of diseases, which also comprises peripheral SpA (including psoriatic arthritis, reactive arthritis and arthropathy of inflammatory bowel disease), and undifferentiated SpA.

IntechOpen

Ankylosing Spondylitis (AS)—the most known and investigated form of SpA—is a chronic, immunomediated arthritis, usually progressive, characterised by inflammation of the axial skeleton, entheses, peripheral joints and extra-articular sites like the eye, bowel and heart. It is also designed as Radiographic axial spondyloarthritis (axSpA). This term comprises the whole group of patients with sacroiliitis (AS or radiographic axSpA) and without radiographic sacroiliitis (non-radiographic axSpA).

Radiographic sacroiliitis has been considered the hallmark of AS but it is a late finding. Patients may complain of back pain for years without any findings in classic X-rays, but MRI shows signs of inflammation much earlier than structural damage. It is known from historical data that patients with end-stage AS were recognised by a stooped posture and by the presence of syndesmophytes on spine X-rays.

The first criteria for use in population surveys to investigate the epidemiology of AS were proposed in Rome in 1961 [17] and revised in New York in 1966 [18]. The Rome criteria were not widely used because the lack of sacroiliitis was considered too greater loss of specificity. These criteria employed new objective clinical methods to measure spinal mobility but sacroiliitis (at least grade 2 bilateral radiographic sacroiliitis) was later introduced in the New York criteria [19]. These diagnostic criteria were modified by van der Linden in 1984 [20], which provided greater specificity and introduced their extension to non-axial spondyloarthropathies.

Because the lone concept of AS was challenged, classification criteria were developed by Amor in 1990 [21], followed by the European Spondyloarthropathy Study Group (ESSG) [22]. More recently in 2004, the Assessment of Spondyloarthritis International Society (ASAS) decided to improve SpA criteria mainly for application in early disease [23]. The ASAS criteria performed better than the Amor and ESSG criteria which were developed in the pre-MRI era, showing that MRI of the axial skeleton was crucial for the characterisation of the SpA. MRI allowed to define two subsets of axial spondyloarthritis (axSpA): non-radiographic axial SpA, and radiographic SpA, considered two stages of the same disease. These new criteria were created to facilitate research in SpA— observational studies and clinical trials, although today they are also used as diagnostic criteria in clinical practice by a large number of rheumatologists.

Metrology, like radiology, contributed significantly to AS characterisation and to research on SpA, and also for evaluating improvements in function and activity in patients subjected to treatments in daily practice or in clinical trials. Lumbar flexion measurements had been used since Schober [24]; Macrae and Wright (1969) [25] introduced the modified Schober index that was judged as a reasonably reliable measure of lumbar flexion. Several other measures were proposed like the tragus-to-wall, the chest expansion, hip mobility involving a goniometer, the intermalleolar distance, the finger-to-floor distance, the C7-to-iliac crest line distraction and the lateral finger-to-floor distance. In 1994, Jenkinson evaluated the metrology results from 20 movements and chose five of them that were collectively named BASMI—the Bath Ankylosing Spondylitis Metrology Index [26]. This index proved to be sensitive to changes in patient mobility, although it had a poor relationship with radiology. It has obvious advantages over radiology because it could be repeated as often as required, is able to be quickly performed and did not require expensive equipment, and most importantly, examines parameters that are not irreversible, unlike radiographic changes.

In the early 1980, the concept of self-administered questionnaires became acceptable to investigate rheumatic diseases. One of these—the Health Assessment Questionnaire (HAQ score) [27]—was designed to evaluate the health status of patients with rheumatoid arthritis, but was modified for use with spondyloarthropathies (HAQ-S) [28]. In 1988, Dougados et al. [29] produced the first functional index designed for patients with AS, followed by Calin A in 1994 with the Bath Ankylosing Spondylitis Functional Index (BASFI) [30], by the validation and development of a Dutch version of the French index (Creemers et al.) [31] and by the Leeds Disability Questionnaire (Abbott et al. 1994) [32]. These questionnaires had all very high Cronbach's alpha scores and were good tools for research on group comparisons and for assessing individual patients in a clinical situation [33]. Another index, designed to evaluate disease activity, was published in 1994 (Garrett et al.) [34]—the Bath Ankylosing Spondylitis Activity Index (BASDAI). This index was considered appropriate as a research tool in group comparisons.

The mechanisms of the pathogenesis of Ankylosing Spondylitis are complex and are not completely recognised. During the last years, several studies established the high heritability of the disease. One of them, the UK Biobank study [35], used the Affymetrix Axiom chip and the hereditability was estimated at 69.1%. The International AS Genetics Consortium Study using the Illumina Immunochip estimated hereditability at 32.7% [36]. Further to genetic factor, there are other factors that may be associated with the disease pathogenesis—environmental factors, altered mucosal immunity, altered gut microbiome, disregulation of the immune system and factors associated with the axial and peripheral skeleton and enthesis. HLA-B*27 is possibly the strongest genetic association with AS and is remarkably polymorphic. To date, at least 271 subtypes have been reported, some of them not disease associated, and the ancestral subtype is suggested to be HLA-B*27:05 that is present in nearly all populations [37]. Several other major histocompatibility complex (MHC) alleles were identified in AS negative HLA-B*27, some of them conferring protection. HLAB*60 was the first to be associated with AS B*27 negative patients [38]. The non-MHC genetic associations were identified through genome-wide association studies (GWAS). The first AS GWAS, the Wellcome Trust Case Control Consortium (WTCCC) and the Australo-Anglo-American Spondylitis Consortium (2007), identified single nucleotide polymorphisms (SNPs) in endoplasmic reticulum aminopeptidase 1 (ERAP1) and interleukin 23 receptor (IL23R) [39]. Other GWAS identified new AS susceptibility loci that can be classified into categories: cytokines and cytokine receptors, mucosal immunity factors, M1-aminopeptidases, transcription factors and intergenic regions. These groups of loci may then be divided mainly into two pathways—the interleukin 23/interleukin 17A (IL-23/IL-17A) and the tumour necrosis factor (TNF) genes [40]. Some of these susceptibility genes identified in these pathways were explored as targets for AS treatment. The successful development of drugs targeting IL-23/Il-17 axis for diseases associated with IL-23/IL-17A illustrates the great value of genetics in drug development.

2. Conclusion

Ankylosing Spondylitis is a fascinating disease that since its first description in 1691–1695 has been the object of an intense research across the world. Several groups focused their research on different aspects of AS: epidemiology, diagnostic criteria, metrology, functional indexes, radiology, genetics and therapy.

All these areas of research gave important contributions to the updated knowledge of AS, although several mechanisms that may help to explain the disease pathogenesis are still unknown. Relevant breakthroughs were obtained through genome-wide association studies (GWAS) with the identification of genes and pathways involved in susceptibility or protection. These advances on the knowledge of AS were crucial and allowed the development of new treatments which modified significantly the disease prognosis.

Author details

Jácome Bruges Armas[1,2]

1 Epidemiology and Molecular Biology Service (SEEBMO), Hospital de Santo Espirito de Angra do Heroísmo, Terceira Island, The Azores, Portugal

2 Comprehensive Health Research Centre (CHRC), Nova Medical School, University of Lisbon, Lisbon, Portugal

*Address all correspondence to: brugesarmas@gmail.com

References

[1] Strumpell A. Lehrbuch der speziellen Pathologie und Therapie der inneren Krankheiten. Vol. 2. Leipzig: Gogel; 1884. p. 457

[2] Strumpell A. Bemerkung über die chronische ankylosierende Entzündung der Wirbelsäule und der Hüftgelenke. Deutsche Zeitschrift für. Nervenheilkunde. 1897;**11**:338

[3] von Bechterew W. Steifigkeit der Wirbelsäule und ihre Verkrümmung als besondere Erkrankungsform. Neurologisches Zentralblatt. 1893;**12**:426

[4] von Bechterew W. Über ankylosierende Entzündung der Wirbelsäule und der grossen Extremitätengelenke. Deutsche Zeitschrift für Nervenheilkunde. 1899;**15**:37

[5] Marie P. Sur la Spondylose rhizomélique. Revue de Médicine. 1898;**18**:285

[6] Léri L. La spondylose rhizomelique. Revue de Medicine. 1899;**19**:597 La spondylose rhizomelique. Ibid, 1899: 690. La spondylose rhizomelique. Ibid, 1899: 801

[7] Léri L. Études sur les Affections de la Colunne Vertebrale. Paris: Masson; 1926

[8] Krebs W. Zur Frage der sogenannten rheumatischen Erkrankungen der Wirbelsäule. Deutsche Medizinische Wochenschrift. 1930;**56**:220-270

[9] Bachmann A. Ein Beitrag zur Spondylarthritis ankylopoietica. Fortschritte auf dem Gebiete der Röntgenstrahlen. 1930;**42**:500

[10] Buckley CW. Spondylitis deformans. British Medical Journal. 1931;**1**:1108

[11] Scott SG. Chronic infection of the sacroiliac joint as a possible cause of spondylitis adolescents. Br J Radiology. 1936;**9**:126

[12] Reiter H. Über eine bisher anerkannte spirochäten Infektion (Spirochaetosis arthritica). Deutsche Medizinische Wochenschrift. 1916;**42**:1535

[13] Schlosstein L, Terasaki PI, Bluestone R, Pearson CM. High association of an HL-A antigen, W27, with ankylosing spondylitis. The New England Journal of Medicine. 1973;**288**:704

[14] Brewerton DR, Caffrey H, Hart FR, James DCO, Nicholls A, Sturrock R. Ankylosing spondylitis and HLA 27. Lancet. 1973;**1**:904

[15] De Blecourt J. Hereditary factors in rheumatoid arthritis and ankylosing spondylitis. In: The Epidemiology of Chronic Rheumatism. Vol. 1. Oxford: Blackwell; 1963. p. 258

[16] Robinson HS, Gofton JP, Price GE. A study of rheumatic diseases in a Canadian Indian population. Annals of the Rheumatic Diseases. 1963;**22**:232

[17] Kellgren JH, Jeffrey MR, Ball J, (eds). The Epidemiology of Chronic Rheumatism. Vol. 1. Oxford: Blackwell; 1963. p. 326

[18] Bennett PH, Burch TA. Wood. In: Population Studies of the Rheumatic Diseases. Amsterdam: Excerpta Medica Foundation; 1968. p. 456

[19] Moll JMH, Wright V. New York clinical criteria for ankylosing spondylitis. Annals of the Rheumatic Diseases. 1973;**32**:354-363

[20] van der Linden SM, Valkenberg HÁ, Cats A. Evaluation of diagnostic criteria for ankylosing spondylitis. A proposal for the modification of the New York criteria. Arthritis and Rheumatism. 1984;**27**:361-368

[21] Amor B, Dougados M, Mijiyawa M. Criteria for the classification of spondyloarthopathies. Revue du Rhumatisme et des Maladies Ostéo-Articulaires. 1990;**57**:85-89

[22] Dougados M, van der Linden S, Jublin R, et al. The European Spondyloarthropathy study group preliminary criteria for the classification of spondyloarthropathy. Arthritis and Rheumatism. 1991;**34**:1218-1227

[23] Rudwaleit M, van der Heijde D, Landewé R, Listing J, et al. The development of assessment of Spondylo arthritis international society classification criteria for axial spondyloarthritis (part II): Validation and final selection. Annals of the Rheumatic Diseases. 2009;**68**:777-783

[24] Schober von P. The lumbar vertebral column and backache. Münchener Medizinische Wochenschrift. 1937;**84**:336-338

[25] Macrae IF, Wright V. Measurement of back movement. Annals of the Rheumatic Diseases. 1969;**28**:584-589

[26] Jenkinson TR, Mallorie PA, Whitelock HC, Kennedy LG, Garrett SL, Calin A. Defining spinal mobility in ankylosing spondylitis. The Bath ankylosing spondylitis disease activity index. The Journal of Rheumatology. 1994;**21**:1694-1698

[27] Fries JF, Spitz P, Kraines RG, Holman HR. Measurement of patient outcome in arthritis. Arthritis and Rheumatism. 1980;**23**:137-145

[28] Daltroy LH, Larson MG, Roberts WN, Liang MH. A modification of the health assessment questionnaire for the spondyloarthropathies. The Journal of Rheumatology. 1990;**17**:946-950

[29] Dougados M, Gueguen A, Nakache J-P, Nguyen M, Amor B. Evaluation of a functional index and an articular index in ankylosing spondylitis. The Journal of Rheumatology. 1988;**15**:302-307

[30] Calin A, Garrett SL, Whitelock HC, et al. A new approach to defining functional ability in ankylosing spondylitis: The development of the Bath ankylosing spondylitis functional index. The Journal of Rheumatology. 1994;**21**:2281-2285

[31] Creemers MCW, Van't Hof MA, MJAM F, de Putte LBA V, FWJ G, PLCM VR. A Dutch version of the functional index for ankylosing spondylitis: Development and validation in a long-term study. British Journal of Rheumatology. 1994;**33**:842-846

[32] Abbott CA, Helliwell PS, Chamberlain MA. Functional assessment in ankylosing spondylitis: Evaluation of a new self-administered questionnaire and correlation with anthropometric variables. British Journal of Rheumatology. 1994;**33**:1060-1066

[33] Jones S. Life-assurance investigation results. In: Ankylosing Spondylitis. London: NASS Newsletter; 1994. pp. 5-6

[34] Garrett SL, Jenkinson TR, Kennedy LG, Whitelock HC, Gaisford P, Calin A. A new approach to defining disease status in ankylosing spondylitis: The Bath ankylosing spondylitis activity index. The Journal of Rheumatology. 1994;**21**:277-281

[35] Available from: http://www.nealelab.is/blog/2017/9/15/

heritability-of-2000-traits-and-disorders-in-the-uk-biobank.

[36] Ellinghaus D, Jostins L, Spain SL, Cortes A, Bethune J, Han B, et al. Analysis of five chronic inflammatory diseases identifies 27 new associations and highlights disease-specific patterns at shared loci. Nature Genetics. 2016;**48**(5):510-518

[37] Li Z, Brown MA. Progress of genome-wide association studies of ankylosing spondylitis. Clinical Translational Immunology. 1 Dec 2017;**6**(12):e163. DOI: 10.1038/cti.2017.49

[38] Brown MA, Pile KD, Kennedy LG, Calin A, Darke C, Bell J, et al. HLA class I associations of ankylosing spondylitis in the white population in the United Kingdom. Annals of the Rheumatic Diseases. Apr 1996;**55**(4):268-270. DOI: 10.1136/ard.55.4.268

[39] Wellcome Trust Case Control C Australo-Anglo_American Spondylitis C, Burton PR, Clayton DG, Cardon LR, Craddock N, et al. Association scan of 14500 nonsynonymous SNPs in four diseases identifies autoimmunity variants. Nature Genetics. 2007;**39**:1329-1337

[40] Brown MA, Wordsworth PB. Genetics in ankylosing spondylitis – Current state of the art and translation into clinical outcomes. Best Practice & Research Clinical Rheumatology. 2018;**31**(6):763-776. DOI: 10.1016/j.berh.2018.09.005

Chapter 2

Diagnostic/Classification Criteria

Razvan Adrian Ionescu, Horatiu Popoviciu and Florentin Ananu Vreju

Abstract

Diagnostic criteria are used, as the name suggests, to make diagnosis of disease. They should encompass those characteristics that we find in every patient with the disease they are designed for. Therefore, it is extremely difficult to design such criteria. Classification criteria, on the other hand, are intended to be used only in already diagnosed patients, to classify them as having the respective disease, mainly for research purposes. Nevertheless, since classification criteria encompass those characteristics of the disease that are present in the majority of patients, it is only natural to try to use them as a helping tool in the diagnostic endeavor. This should be done appropriately, bearing in mind that the patient not fulfilling every one of them, can and may be still diagnosed as having ankylosing spondylitis, even though he/she cannot be classified as such. Classification criteria for ankylosing spondylitis (AS) have changed over time, due to the new insight obtained into the pathogenic mechanisms of the disease. Moreover, a patient fulfilling them is sometimes the initial step mandated by the paying authorities for reimbursement of therapies. All these reasons and others highlight the need to understand the different facets of the diagnostic/classification criteria and their best use.

Keywords: diagnostic criteria, classification criteria, ankylosing spondylitis, spondylarthritis, imaging, HLA B27

1. Introduction

In order to treat patients, a doctor, regardless of his/her specialty, must establish a diagnosis. The task of establishing a correct diagnosis can sometimes be very difficult. In such a circumstance, the existence of a set of diagnostic criteria makes the task easier. On the other hand, in order to establish a set of criteria that can be called "diagnostic criteria," each used item must be present in every patient with the disease. That is what makes defining a set of items as diagnostic criteria extremely difficult. When the clinical, biological, and imagistic pictures of a disease are very variable, such is the case with ankylosing spondylitis, this process is even more complicated.

With the medical technological development characterizing the last 30–40 years, new pathogenic mechanisms have been unveiled, and it became evident that new characteristics of disease may be used as items to classify or, even, diagnose our patients.

Diagnostic/classification criteria are extremely useful in daily clinical practice, especially when the clinical picture of a certain patient is not "clear-cut." In such a circumstance, checking for the items that make a diagnosis/classification criterion might be of value in that it might help review the clinical aspects that are part of the entire clinical spectrum of a disease and establish if the patient's "fit" into the criteria. Fortunately, we have professional associations that do the entire process of establishing sets of criteria for diseases, so that we can use them for our patients.

2. Diagnostic/classification criteria: are they the same?

Diagnostic criteria, as their name implies, are used to make a diagnosis. This means they should contain those specific items that a doctor can find in ALL patients with a certain disease. So, any characteristic of that disease (should it be a clinical or laboratory or imaging one) that is NOT present in ALL patients cannot be a diagnostic criterion. As a consequence, diagnostic criteria should be infallible, unfailing to make the right diagnosis. But let us, clinicians, be realistic: for how many of the characteristics of a diseases can we say that is present in ALL our patients, to define it like a diagnostic criterion?! And this is also true for non-clinical items, as well.

This became more evident with technological progress that allowed us to get deeper into pathogenic processes and acknowledge the fact that a finding (of any nature) is seldom pathognomonic for a disease or a diagnosis. Moreover, the exponential development of clinical research (i.e., randomized control trials) made it extremely necessary to apply interventions (mainly therapeutic) to as homogeneous as possible patient populations.

Hence, the need to define criteria that would encompass disease characteristics (clinical or non-clinical) that are found in the MAJORITY of patients that we encounter in clinical daily practice and not necessarily in ALL of them. These are classification criteria. They should be used, as per their name, just to classify, not to diagnose, patients. That means that they should be applied ONLY to already diagnosed patients. So, they should NOT be used for diagnosing people with diseases, but to classify patients already diagnosed. Classifying diagnosed patients according to certain criteria is very practical when we want to compare different treatments in a population with a disease, because, as aforementioned, this is a very good way to ensure homogeneity of compared populations.

Classification criteria are, therefore, used for research purposes (comparing different interventions in already diagnosed homogeneous populations), while diagnostic criteria are used for making a diagnosis in an individual patient.

In daily clinical practice, things are not that clear-cut. Actually, the majority of rheumatologists use classification criteria established for certain rheumatological diseases, for diagnostic purposes, as well as for research purposes. And this is not wrongdoing, in the sense that, reviewing the most frequently encountered characteristics of a disease might prove very useful in trying to diagnose an individual. And there is no doubt that!

Problems arise only when a physician does not diagnose a disease in an individual only because this individual does not fulfill the classification criteria, even though there are some other characteristics that would enable a more open-minded physician to make that right diagnosis. Probably one of the best examples in this respect pertains to the 1982 American College of Rheumatology (ACR) classification criteria and the 2019 European Ligue Against Rheumatism (EULAR)/ACR classification criteria for systemic lupus erythematosus [1, 2]: in the first set of criteria, low levels of complement had no place, even though very many patients would have such levels; so, if one was using the 1982 set of classification criteria in order to make a diagnosis of a certain patient, one would potentially be missing those patients that did not fulfill four criteria, even if they would have low complement levels. Of course, over time, as our knowledge of diseases increases, classification criteria evolve according to the need of diagnosing as many patients as possible, as early as possible, in order to treat them the most early possible, to prevent complications and disability for our patients.

3. Diagnostic/classification criteria in ankylosing spondylitis

3.1 Modified New York criteria

Ankylosing spondylitis is a more than 100-year-old disease, characterized by bone formation as a result of inflammation of entheseal sites across the body. The inflammatory nature of this disease has consequences on other systems and organs in the body, than the musculoskeletal system, leading to extra-articular manifestations of the disease. These may consistently add to the morbidity and mortality of AS. This emphasizes on the need to establish a correct diagnosis as soon as possible.

To this day, there are no specific lab tests for diagnosing AS [3]. Moreover, even if usually, in inflammatory/autoimmune disease, the patient has elevated levels of blood markers of inflammation (erythrocyte sedimentation rate [ESR] and C-reactive protein [CRP]), a lot of patients with AS may have active disease with normal levels of inflammatory markers [4]. To further complicate the matter, even the most encountered serologic marker of AS, that is, HLA-B27, is absent in up to 30% of patients [5, 6], while its prevalence in the general population is around 6–10% [5]; furthermore, only about 10% of individuals having positive HLA-B27 will ever develop AS [7]. Remember, all this information is long time known.

Now, bearing in mind all of this, it is quite conceivable that, to this day, in the absence of a set of diagnostic criteria, we still use the "modified New York classification criteria" to help us diagnose ankylosing spondylitis. These criteria are depicted in **Table 1** [modified from 8].

We very well know that the most prominent clinical feature of AS is inflammatory back pain [3]. Unfortunately, as knowledge evolved, we realized that the pathogenic process of AS starts long before the clinical diagnosis is established, so there is a consistent diagnostic gap, between the occurrence of the inflammatory back pain and the moment the patient receives the diagnosis of AS. This is, at least partially, due to the radiological criterion in the modified New York criteria. And that is because of the definitions of the different grades of sacroiliitis. They are defined in **Table 2** (modified from [3]). As one can see, looking at those definitions, it is quite difficult to make a clear-cut difference between the different grades of sacroiliitis, but especially between grade 2 and grade 1 or 3. This is mainly due to the particular spatial orientation of the sacroiliac joint, which is oblique. That "special" orientation precludes a good visualization of the entire sacroiliac joint on a standard posteroanterior radiograph of the pelvis [3]. In trying to overcome this issue, one may use the Ferguson view, which consists of the rotation of the pelvis 30 degrees, thus getting the sacroiliac joint perpendicular into the way of the X-ray beam [9].

Another way to try to overcome the problem of the sacroiliac joint spatial orientation is to perform X-ray examination on each sacroiliac joint at a time [10]. Let alone

1. Radiological criterion

   Bilateral sacroiliitis grade at least II or unilateral sacroiliitis grade III or IV

2. Clinical criteria

   a. Low back pain associated to stiffness of at least 3 months duration that is improved by exercise and is not relieved by rest

   b. Limitation of range of motion of the lumbar spine both in the sagittal and the frontal plane

   c. Limitation of chest expansion relative to values normal for age and gender

Definite AS is diagnosed if the radiological criterion plus two of the three clinical criteria are present in the patient.

Table 1.
Modified New York classification criteria for ankylosing spondylitis.

Grade	Definition
0	Normal
1	Suspiciously abnormal
2	Subchondral bone sclerosis, possible some erosions
3	Pseudo enlargement of the joint space, severe erosions
4	Complete ankylosis

Table 2.
Radiographic grading of sacroiliitis.

that there is no evidence that this kind of approach is superior to the standard pelvic X-ray approach [10], performing the standard radiograph of the pelvis may add some important clues to the diagnosis of AS: it captures the last lumbar vertebrae, allowing to search for the "vertebral squaring" sign (consequence of the vertebral osseous inflammation) [11] and it, also, captures the coxo-femural joints, allowing to visualize their frequent involvement in AS [3].

Regardless of these considerations, using the modified New York classification criteria for making a diagnosis of AS will be totally useless for early AS, since it takes a lot of time (sometimes as long as 10 years) for the aforementioned findings to become apparent on an X-ray [12, 13]. This is of great concern, because, by the time the sacroiliac joints radiograph exhibits bilateral grade II sacroiliitis, the spine (as well as other joints) of the patient may be already fused, not to mention the possible occurrence during that time, of extra-articular manifestations of the disease, a situation that makes treatment much more difficult.

This has led to the use of other imaging techniques to try to visualize more early the pathological processes involved in AS. Thus, computed tomography (CT) and magnetic resonance imaging (MRI) were tried to image AS, and it was found that CT is superior to MRI when it comes to visualize the chronic bony changes [10]. On the other hand, MRI is a technique that allows the visualization of both chronic (structural) lesions and acute (inflammatory) ones. Now we know that the way to imaging bone marrow edema (that is, osseous inflammation in its most active form), which is the most suggestive pathological imaging finding for ankylosing spondylitis, is by using MRI [14]. Moreover, MRI is capable of visualizing early changes at the level of the cartilage as well [15] and does not expose the patient to radiation Thus, the use of MRI helped defining the two subsets of axial spondylarthritis (ax SpA):

non-radiographic ax SpA (that is, the axial spondylarthritis that does not fulfill the radiographic criterion of the modified New York criteria) and radiographic ax SpA (that is, the axial spondylarthritis that does fulfill the radiographic criterion of the modified New York criteria, which is in fact AS). These two subsets are considered two stages of the same disease [15].

3.2 ASAS classification criteria

The evidence that the modified New York criteria fail to detect early AS and that MRI helps visualize early bone marrow edema led to the development of a new set of criteria: the ASAS classification criteria. They were developed and published in 2009, by the Assessment of SpondyloArthritis international Society (ASAS) group [16]. You can view those to be used for axial spondylarthritis in **Figure 1**.

Remember, this is a set of classification, not diagnostic criteria, even though both diagnosis and classification processes operate with the same set of parameters [15].

The most important first thing that one should consider when applying criteria is to know the population to which they are applicable. In this respect, the ASAS classification criteria for ax SpA should be used only in patients with back pain of at least 3 months duration, which started before the age of 45. Why is that? On the one hand, because AS is a disease that starts, in most cases, in the third or fourth decade of life [15] and, on the other hand, because 45 years of age is a good milestone to consider when considering a diagnosis of AS, in the primary care setting [17]. In most cases, the back pain will be low back pain, but some patients will have other localization of the back pain. Some characteristics of the pain will make it more susceptible to be an inflammatory pain, and this, in turn, will raise the probability of the patient having ax SpA, to around 30% based only on no other clinical feature than pain [18].

There have been multiple proposals for items that would enable a doctor to classify back pain as inflammatory back pain; historically, the oldest set of criteria (1977) is that of Calin et al. [19], who upon studying 42 patients with AS and 21 with mechanical low back pain, concluded that a patient fulfilling four of the following: age at onset lower than 40 years, duration of back pain more than 3 months,

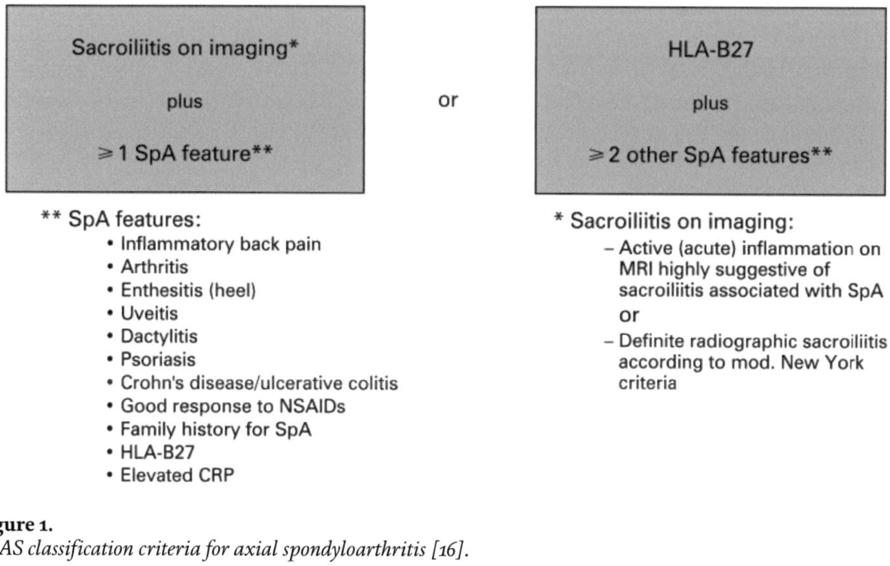

Figure 1.
ASAS classification criteria for axial spondyloarthritis [16].

insidious onset, morning stiffness and improvement with exercise can be classified as having inflammatory back pain. Then, we had the modified Berlin criteria for inflammatory back pain proposed by Rudwaleit et al. [20], who, based on the study of 101 AS patients and 112 patients with mechanical back pain, stated that inflammatory back pain may be assumed in a patient with chronic back pain with onset before the age of 45 if the patient has two of the following: morning stiffness more than 30 minute, improvement of the pain with exercise and not with rest, alternating buttock pain or awakening at second part of night because of the pain. Finally, in 2009, Sieper et al. [21] published the ASAS criteria for inflammatory back pain, which encompass the following items: age of onset of the pain less than 40 years, an insidious onset, the improvement of the pain with exercise and no improvement with rest and the existence of pain at night, with improvement upon getting up. Based on evaluating 648 patients with chronic back pain, if four out of the five aforementioned items are present, then the patient has inflammatory back pain with a sensitivity of 79.6% and a specificity of 72.4% [21]. These values might seem small, but they enable a physician to ascertain a patient as having inflammatory back pain as a first step to take on the road to establishing a correct diagnosis of radiographic ax SpA.

After properly selecting the population on which to apply the criteria, physicians have two alternative pathways to take ("arms") to classify patients as ax SpA (radiographic or non-radiographic): the "imaging arm" and the "HLA arm."

If the patient has sacroiliitis on imaging, then the doctor needs only one additional SpA feature to classify the patient. Noteworthy, it does not matter what imaging method we use; it could be either MRI showing acute active inflammation highly suggestive of sacroiliitis (in this case, we are talking about non-radiographic SpA) or an X-ray showing definite radiographic sacroiliitis according to modified New York criteria (in which case we are talking about radiographic SpA or AS) [16].

If no imaging technique is available, one can use the "HLA" arm: one should look for the presence of HLA-B27 positivity in their patient and, if so, seek for at least two more SpA features. The SpA features considered (**Table 3**) are either clinical and laboratory signs of skeletal or extra-skeletal inflammatory involvement (inflammatory back pain, arthritis, enthesitis, dactylitis, uveitis, psoriasis, Chron's colitis, good response to NSAIDs, elevated CRP) or familial history and B27 positivity [16].

It is noteworthy that peripheral involvement, extra-articular involvement, as well as response to medication, are incorporated in the axial SpA criteria, thus emphasizing on the importance of exploring all these characteristics of the disease, since they are all relevant for the diagnosis as well as for the classification of these patients. Just for example, the specificity of heel enthesitis for ax SpA is around 90% and that of dactylitis around 96% [15]. When it comes to extra-articular manifestations of SpA, the most frequent (around 20%) and potentially extremely damaging is acute anterior uveitis, followed by psoriasis (around 10%) and inflammatory bowel disease (2–7%) [15].

The ASAS classification criteria, all together, have a specificity of 84.4% and a sensitivity of 82.9% [16], which is quite good. When using the imaging criteria alone, the sensibility falls to 66.2%, but the specificity rises to 97.3% [16], which means that if the imaging criteria are negative, we might miss a few patients, but if they are positive, we are (almost) certain that we are doing the right classification for a particular patient. Moreover, this very high specificity of this set of criteria provides great confidence for the practitioner who finds them positive, even in the diagnosis making process, not only in the classification process.

Inflammatory back pain
Arthritis
Enthesitis
Dactylitis
Uveitis
Psoriasis
Crohn's disease/ulcerative colitis
Good response to NSAID's
HLA B27
Family history
Elevated CRP

Table 3.
SpA features (modified from [16]).

The development of the ASAS classification criteria for axial SpA really represented a major step forward, first because of their potential to correctly discover patients in an early stage of their disease. Since the primarily objective of any treatment for rheumatic inflammatory diseases is avoidance of structural damage, and this can be done only if we "intercept" the patient's disease as early as possible (that is, before the disease has already produced its deleterious effects), having a way to identify patients in that early stage of their disease is crucial to the successfulness of any therapy. Moreover, even if their specificity and sensibility are not 100%, the development of the ASAS classification criteria really stimulated research in the field of spondyloarthropathies, which in turn allowed medicine to better understand the pathogenesis, course, and prognosis of that group of diseases [22].

3.3 Making the diagnosis of ankylosing spondylitis

Even if, as mentioned above, the use the same set of parameters [15] and, even though this does not always happen in clinical daily practice, the diagnostic approach of ankylosing spondylitis should be different from the classification approach, because of several reasons [15].

First of all, the aim of the two processes is different: while classification aims at defining as homogeneous as possible population, for research purposes, diagnosing is establishing what is the disease that the patient presents, in daily routine practice [15].

Then, when making a diagnosis (and not only for ankylosing spondylitis), we always take into consideration a differential, which is not the case when classifying a patient [15]. The whole process of diagnosing a patient relies on many different tests that have a pre-test probability and a positive and negative likelihood ratio; their values vary depending on several factors (the test itself, background populations, etc.). This does not happen with the classification process, which uses only those tests that are part of the classification items and only with the "present" or "absent" value (since the whole classification process depends on the presence or absence of the criteria). This "yes" or "no" approach is also valuable for the outcome of the classification approach, and that is different from the outcome of the diagnostic assessment that has as outcome the probability of the presence of disease [15].

To summarize, when we make the diagnosis of ankylosing spondylitis, we should use the classification items just to remember which are the disease characteristics that we find most often in such patients and not to confirm or exclude disease. In other words, if a practitioner tries to diagnose a patient's disease, the fact that the patient does not fulfill the classification criteria for AS does not mean that the patient does not have AS. If the practitioner finds enough reasons to diagnose the patient as having AS, even if the patient cannot be classified as having AS, then, the patient has AS and the practitioner will be able to sustain his opinion to anyone. It is just like such a patient will be in the group that does have AS, but not have all of the most common characteristics of AS.

So, the two processes, the two approaches are completely different and should be used accordingly in the care of patients with AS.

4. Use of diagnostic/classification criteria in ankylosing spondylitis

In the absence of diagnostic criteria for ankylosing spondylitis, the diagnostic approach toward a patient's disease is sometimes difficult and complicated. Thus, to make their life easier, it would seem quite normal and at hand for doctors to use the classification criteria for diagnosis as well, even though, as pointed out earlier, this is not conceptually correct or appropriate. Being aware of that "psychological flaw," it is very interesting to try and find out what is the situation in the real-life setting: what is the attitude of practitioners around the world toward using the existing classification criteria (modified New York and ASAS)?!

To answer this question, Rich-Garg and coworkers [23] designed and carried out a study among rheumatologists in five countries on four continents. There were 478 rheumatologists that participated in this survey regarding multiple aspects of the modified New York criteria for AS and ASAS criteria for ax SpA and their use. The mean age of participants was around 50 so, on an average, they were quite experienced rheumatologists, and 31% were females; 90% of respondents declared spending more than 75% of their time in clinical practice [23].

The survey showed that two-thirds of the responding rheumatologists "usually or always" use the ASAS classification criteria to make the diagnosis of ax SpA [23]. This is somehow expected (because using the criteria, sometimes "makes life easier") and somehow unexpected (because one would expect that experienced rheumatologists would use the criteria just "sometimes"). Anyway, using the criteria for diagnosis, in real-life daily clinical practice, can lead to over-diagnosis [24], which in turn can lead to over-treatment, which can have potentially negative consequences. Another important finding resulting from this survey is the fact that doctors having completed rheumatology training more recently were more likely to use the classification criteria for diagnostic purposes [23]! This highlights the need for reinforcing the difference between diagnostic and classification approach to rheumatologists in training, who should be able, by the time they complete their specialty training, to use them appropriately.

Another interesting finding of the aforementioned study [23] is the perception of the specificity for diagnosing ax SpA, of the various SpA features. Inflammatory back pain, a totally subjective finding, which is the cornerstone for using the classification criteria, was thought very specific for ax SpA diagnosis by 44% of rheumatologists [23]. In contrast with this, the quite objective items such as enthesitis and peripheral inflammatory arthritis were thought very specific for ax SpA diagnosis by just 39%

and 25% of respondents, respectively [23]. Bearing in mind that the actual specificity of heel enthesitis is around 90% [15], this finding of the survey is rather surprising and might point to the fact that many rheumatologists are not aware of the real importance of enthesitis in the diagnosis of ax SpA; this may also have to do with the fact that, in the classification criteria, the various items do not differ in specific importance.

When exploring the use of imaging in the real-life diagnosing approach by rheumatologists, the survey [23] found that the majority of respondents use the X-ray of the sacroiliac joints as the initial imaging assessment modality [23]. This was to be expected since the access to radiology services is more widespread than that to other imaging modalities. On the other hand, the use of the X-ray assessment of sacroiliac joints might occasionally lose some patients, because there is a wide temporal gap between the first symptom of AS and the first abnormality found on the X-ray assessment. This might also be one of the explanations of the fact that the majority of rheumatologists rely on themselves to interpret the X-rays [23]. As was to be expected, if the radiographic examination of the sacroiliac joints is normal, most rheumatologists rather order a magnetic resonance imaging study than a computed tomography study [23], to view the potentially existing inflammatory lesions. This approach was to be expected since computed tomography, on the one hand, bears the burden of irradiation and, on the other hand, is not as sensitive for edema as magnetic resonance imaging.

5. Conclusions

Diagnostic criteria and classification criteria are not at all the same thing; they differ conceptually, even if they operate with the same set of items. Their differences make the use of ones instead of the others, totally inappropriate. Moreover, using classification criteria for diagnosing purposes could lead to over-diagnosis, which in turn may have negative consequences. On the other hand, knowing the classification criteria may help and ease the diagnostic process, since they represent the most frequently encountered characteristics of the disease. In daily clinical practice, a great number of rheumatologists use classification criteria for the diagnosis of ankylosing spondylitis and axial spondyloarthritis.

Conflict of interest

The authors declare no conflict of interest.

Author details

Razvan Adrian Ionescu[1], Horatiu Popoviciu[2] and Florentin Ananu Vreju[3*]

1 Colentina Clinical Hospital, Romania

2 Targu Mures County Emergency Hospital, Romania

3 Craiova County Emergency Hospital, Romania

*Address all correspondence to: tane67@gmail.com

References

[1] Tan EM, Cohen AS, Fries JF, Masi AT, McShane DJ, Rothfield NF, et al. The 1982 revised criteria for the classification of systemic lupus erythematosus. Arthritis and Rheumatism. 1982;**25**:1271-1277

[2] Aringer M, Costenbader K, Daikh D, et al. 2019 European league against rheumatism/American College of Rheumatology Classification Criteria for systemic lupus erythematosus. Arthritis & Rhematology. 2019;**71**(9):1400-1412. DOI: 10.1002/art.40930

[3] Raychaudhuri SP, Deodhar A. The classification and diagnostic criteria of ankylosing spondylitis. Journal of Autoimmune. 2014;**48-48**:128-133. DOI: 10.1016/jaut2014.01.015

[4] Poddubnyy DA, Rudwaleit M, Listing J, Braun J, Sieper J. Comparison of a high sensitivity and standard C reactive protein measurement in patients with ankylosing spondylitis and non-radiographic axial spondyloarthritis. Annals of the Rheumatic Diseases. 2010;**69**:1338-1341

[5] Rudwaleit M, van der Heijde D, Khan MA, Braun J, Sieper J. How to diagnose axial spondyloarthritis early. Annals of the Rheumatic Diseases. 2004;**63**(5):535

[6] Rudwaleit M, Haibel H, Baraliakos X, Listing J, Märker-Hermann E, Zeidler H, et al. The early disease stage in axial spondyloarthritis: Results from the German spondyloarthritis inception cohort. Arthritis and Rheumatism. 2009;**60**(3):717-727

[7] Reveille JD, Ball EJ, Khan MA. HLA-B27 and genetic predisposing factors in spondyloarthropathies. Current Opinion in Rheumatology. 2001;**13**:265-272

[8] van der Linden S, Valkenburg HA, Cats A. Evaluation of diagnostic criteria for ankylosing spondylitis. A proposal for modification of the New York criteria. Arthritis and Rheumatism. 1984;**27**:361-368

[9] Resnick D, Niwayama G. Ankylosing spondylitis. In: Resnick D, editor. Diag- Nosis of Bone and Joint Disorders. Philadelphia: WB Saunders; 1981. pp. 1040-1102

[10] Braun J, van der Heijde D. Imaging and scoring in ankylosing spondylitis. Best Practice & Research. Clinical Rheumatology. 2002;**16**:573-604

[11] Aufdermaur M. Pathogenesis of square bodies in ankylosing spondylitis. Annals of the Rheumatic Diseases. 1989;**48**:628-631

[12] Khan MA. Thoughts concerning the early diagnosis of ankylosing spondylitis and related diseases. Clinical Experiment in Rheumatology. 2002;**20**(28):S6-S10

[13] Rudwaleit M, Khan MA, Sieper J. The challenge of diagnosis and classification in early ankylosing spondylitis: Do we need new criteria? Arthritis and Rheumatism. 2005;**52**:1000-1008

[14] Yu W, Feng F, Dion E, Yang H, Jiang M, Genant HK. Comparison of radiography, computed tomography and magnetic resonance imaging in the detection of sacroiliitis accompanying ankylosing spondylitis. Skeletal Radiology. 1998;**27**:311-320

[15] Poddubnyy D. Classification *vs* diagnostic criteria: the challenge of diagnosing axial spondyloarthritis. Rheumatology. 2020;**59**:17

[16] Rudwaleit M, van der Heijde D, Landewe R, et al. The development of assessment of SpondyloArthritis international society classification criteria for axial spondyloarthritis (part II): Validation and final selection. Annals of the Rheumatic Diseases. 2009;**68**:777-783

[17] Poddubnyy D, van Tubergen A, Landewe R, Sieper J, van der Heijde D. Development of an ASAS-endorsed recommendation for the early referral of patients with a suspicion of axial spondyloarthritis. Annals of the Rheumatic Diseases. 2015;**74**:1483-1487

[18] Hermann J, Giessauf H, Schaffler G, Ofner P, Graninger W. Early spondyloarthritis: Usefulness of clinical screening. Rheumatology. 2009;**48**:812-816

[19] Calin A, Porta J, Fries JF, Schurman DJ. Clinical history as a screening test for ankylosing spondylitis. Journal of the American Medical Association. 1977;**237**:2613-2614

[20] Rudwaleit M, Metter A, Listing J, et al. Inflammatory back pain in ankylosing spondylitis: A reassessment of the clinical history for application as classification and diagnostic criteria. Arthritis and Rheumatism. 2006;**54**:569-578

[21] Sieper J, Rudwaleit M, Baraliakos X, et al. The Assessment of SpondyloArthritis international Society (ASAS) handbook: A guide to assess spondyloarthritis. Arthritis and Rheumatism. 2009;**68**:ii1-ii44

[22] Proft F, Poddubnyy D. Ankylosing spondylitis and axial spondyloarthritis: Recent insights and impact of new classification criteria. Therapeutic Advances in Musculoskeletal Diseases. 2018;**10**(5-6):129-139

[23] Rich-Garg N, Danve A, Choi D, et al. Assessing rheumatologists' attitudes and utilization of classification criteria for ankylosing spondylitis and axial spondyloarthritis: A global effort. Clinical Rheumatology. 2021;**40**:949-954

[24] Deodhar A. Axial spondyloarthritis criteria and modified NY criteria: Issues and controversies. Clinical Rheumatology. 2014;**33**(6):741-747

Chapter 3

Imaging Ankylosing Spondylitis

Esra Dilsat Bayrak

Abstract

Ankylosing spondylitis (AS) is a chronic inflammatory disease affecting the spine and the sacroiliac joints. AS occurs with the inflammation of the entheses and formation of syndesmophytes and finally sacral and spinal ankylosis. Imaging demonstrates both inflammatory and chronic lesions. Sacroiliitis is the hallmark of the disease. Spinal changes usually take place in advanced stages of the disease. 1984 The Modified New York criteria evaluated for the diagnosis of AS with definite radiological sacroiliitis (bilaterally grade 2 or unilateral grade 3/4 sacroiliitis) on imaging. The Modified New York criteria are well performed in diagnosing the established disease but its sensitivity is too low in early disease identification and leads to a diagnostic delay. So, in 2009 The Assessment in Spondyloarthritis International Society (ASAS) recommended classification criteria for axial spondyloarthritis (axSpA). Patients have sacroiliitis on imaging and ≥1 SpA features (imaging arm) or positive HLA B27 and ≥2 SpA features (clinical arm) are classified as axial SpA. On the imaging arm, either radiographic sacroiliitis according to Modified New York criteria or active inflammation on MRI is required. Imaging is also used for determining extent of disease, monitoring activity and progression of the disease, assessment of the treatment effect, and prognosis in AS patients.

Keywords: ankylosing spondylitis, imaging, conventional radiography, magnetic resonance imaging, computed tomography

1. Introduction

Ankylosing spondylitis (AS) is a chronic inflammatory disease affecting the spine and the sacroiliac joints. Patients with AS show both active inflammatory and structural changes on imaging.

Sacroiliitis, spondylitis, spondylodiscitis and facet joint arthritis are the typical inflammatory manifestations. These inflammatory lesions lead to chronic structural lesions, such as syndesmophytes and ankylosis, in the later stages of the disease [1].

Imaging of the sacroiliac joint plays an important role in AS, since almost all patients with AS do have involvement of the sacroiliac joints. Inflammation of sacroiliac joint on imaging is the hallmark of AS in both diagnosis and classification.

1.1 Anatomy of the sacroiliac joint

The sacroiliac joint (SIJ) lies between the sacrum and the ilium, formed within sacral segments S1, S2 and S3, about 1–2 mm in width and a joint on either side of the sacrum is held together by a fibrous capsule. The bony anatomy is highly variable in size, shape and contour among individuals.

The surface of the SIJ can be divided into three parts, corresponding to the three sacral elements (S1, S2, S3) that participate in the (sacral) auricular surface, terms like ventral, middle and dorsal part. The lower portion of the cranial limb and the caudal limb are synovial in construction, whereas the upper part of the cranial limb is more fibrous [2, 3].

Six types of anatomical variants were defined as: accessory joints, iliosacral complex, bipartite iliac bony plate, crescent-like iliac bony plate, semicircular defects at the sacral or iliac side and ossification centers. Accessory joint is the most common anatomic variant in sacroiliac joint [3].

2. Conventional radiography

2.1 Technical aspects

Conventional radiography (CR) of the sacroiliac joints (SIJs) is the first recommended modality for the diagnosis of AS and is the gold standard for the assessment

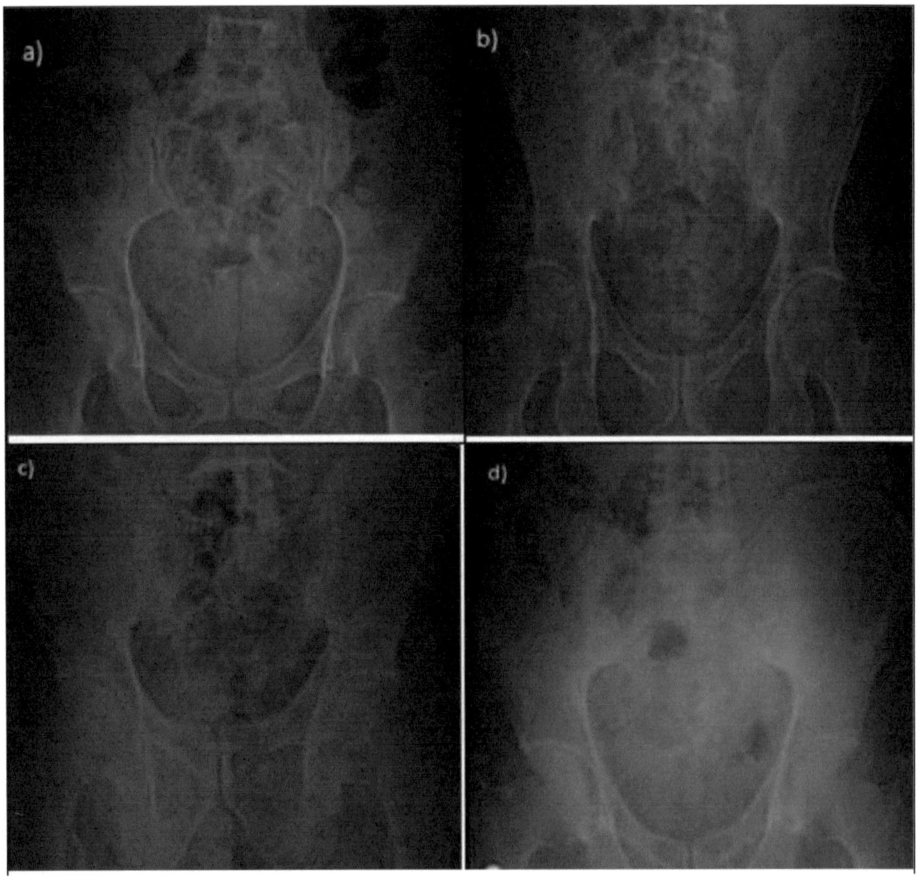

Figure 1.
Grading sacroiliitis according to the New York criteria. a) Grade 1: subtle findings that does not indicate definite AS. b) Grade 2: minimal changes with bilateral small sclerotic areas and erosions on right SIJ. c) Grade 3: bilateral joint narrowing and erosions on right SIJ. d) Grade 4: bilateral total ankylosis.

of structural changes in the spine and SIJs. A frontal projection of the SIJs is preferred. An anterior–posterior view of the SIJs is usually performed with the patient in the supine position [4].

İdeal pelvis AP view should include; entirety of the bony pelvis imaged from superior of the iliac crest to the proximal shaft of the femur, obturator foramina appear symmetrical, iliac wings have an equal concavity and greater trochanters of the proximal femur [5].

2.2 Sacroiliac joint

Typical radiographic findings in the SIJs are erosions, pseudo-widening, sclerosis, bony bridging, and ankylosis. Erosions in the iliac side of the SIJs are the earliest radiographic changes visualized in AS. Definition of diagnostic criteria of radiographic changes of the SIJs has been used according to the 1984 modified New York criteria [6] in AS patients and classification of axSpA according to the 2009 ASAS classification criteria [7].

Grade definition of radiographic changes.

0 Normal.

1 Suspicious changes.

2 Minimal abnormalities: small localized areas with erosion and sclerosis, without alteration in the joint width.

3 Unequivocal abnormality: moderate or advanced sacroiliitis with 1 or more signs of erosions, sclerosis, widening, joint space narrowing, or partial ankylosis.

4 Severe changes: total ankylosis.

According to the modified New York criteria, the radiographic definition of sacroiliitis has a high specificity for axial SpA, but a low sensitivity (30–50%) especially in early disease [8]. Therefore, using only these criteria in the diagnosis of AS may delay the diagnosis of the disease (**Figure 1**).

2.3 Spine

Radiograhic findings of AS patients in the spine are vertebral corner erosions, enthesophytes, vertebral squaring (precursor “shiny corners” seen on x-ray represent circumscribed areas of postinflammatory fatty bone marrow degeneration), sclerosis and erosions of the vertebral endplate, disk calcifications, spondylophytes, syndesmophytes, bony bridging, and/or intervertebral ankylosis and then bamboo spine.

New bone formation, syndesmophytes, and ankylosis of the vertebral column are almost pathognomonic for AS. Syndesmophytes are the best predictors of radiographic progression [9]. Most of the data regarding radiological progression of AS pertains to CR (**Figure 2**) [10].

2.4 Scoring

The most common findings of ankylosing spondylitis in the vertebral column are syndesmophytes and ankylosis. These findings indicate new bone formation, erosions are less common in the vertebral column. Erosion and sclerosis are predictive factors for syndesmophyte formation. Syndesmophyte and ankylosis are best evaluated on conventional radiographs [11, 12]. Syndesmophytes grow and merge and appear as bamboo spine in advanced disease [13]. Radiograhic grading and scoring help us to evaluate the disease activity and progression.

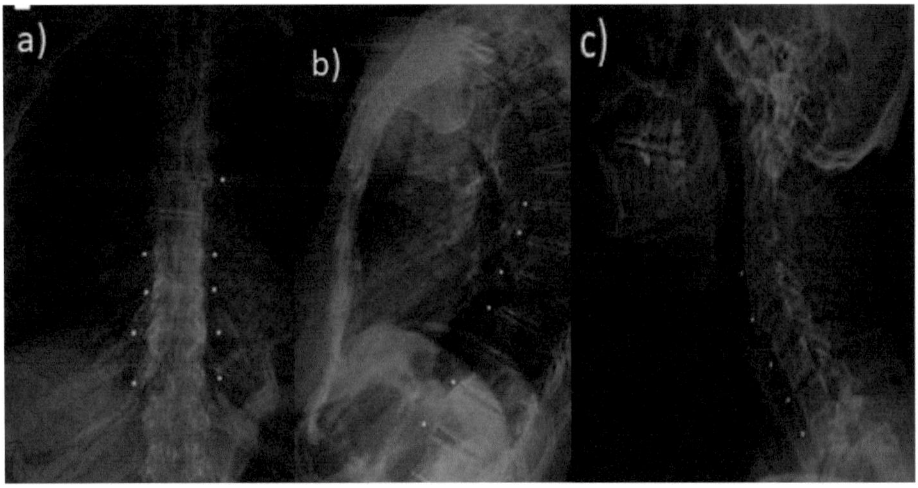

Figure 2.
Radiographs of spine in AS. a)AP view of thoracolumbar vertebrae:extensive syndesmophytes leading bamboo spine b)lateral view demonstrating syndesmophytes c) lateral view of cervical spine: vertical syndesmophytes bridging the anterior vertebral corners.

To date, there are two accepted scoring systems using conventional radiography in AS patients; SASSS/mSASSS [14] and BASRI scores [15].

2.4.1 Modified stoke ankylosing spondylitis spinal score (mSASSS)

mSASSS derived from sum of scores for lumbar spine and cervical spine (range 0–72)

- nominal scoring system used for each site
    - 0 = no abnormality
    - 1 = erosion, sclerosis, or squaring
    - 2 = syndesmophyte
    - 3 = total bony bridging

lumbar sites were lower border of 12th thoracic vertebra, all 5 lumbar vertebrae, and upper boarder of sacrum.

cervical sites were lower border of second cervical vertebra up to and including upper border of first thoracic vertebra; third cervical vertebra scored for erosions and sclerosis, but not squaring.

2.4.2 BASRI

For the lumbar spine, examine both the anteroposterior and lateral radiographs together. The score for the lumbar spine is a composite of the two views. For the cervical spine lateral view is scored.

Score	Grade	Lumbar and cervical spine (grade each as 0–4)
0	Normal	No change
1	Suspicious	No definite change
2	Mild	Any number of erosions, squaring or sclerosis with/without syndesmophytes on ≤2 vertebrae
3	Moderate	Syndesmophytes on ≥3 vertebrae with/without fusion involving 2 vertebrae
4	Severe	Fusion involving ≥3 vertebrae

A modification has been accepted and called BASRI-s for the spine only, BASRI-h for the hips only, and BASRI-t for the summation of both [16].

A study comparing three of these methods (i.e. BASRI, SASSS and mSASSS) concluded that mSASSS is the most appropriate method by which to score radiographic progression in AS [17]. mSASSS is the preferred scoring method for radiographic progression in AS.

2.5 Radiographic progression

According to the definition of mSASSS, radiographic damage is defined as more than 2 points change from baseline [18]. This means that at least 1 new syndesmophyte is formed. This change can be evaluated as improvement or worsening depending on the emergence or disappearance of the new lesion. Definite radiographic damage at baseline is a prognostic factor associated with continuing radiographic progression over time, possibly independent of treatment.

3. Magnetic resonance imaging

Magnetic resonance imaging (MRI) can detect both active inflammatory and structural lesions and capable of detecting both bone marrow edema (BME) or osteitis and erosions before CR [19]. Therefore, MRI is particularly useful for the early diagnosis of AS.

Also, patients with signs or symptoms indicative of SpA but not have structural lesions on conventional radiography, MRI can detect active- chronic lesions for sacroiliitis or spondylitis. These patients can be classified as having 'axial non-radiographic spondyloarthritis (nr-axSpA)' according to criteria developed by the Assessment of Spondyloarthritis International Society (ASAS) [7]. So, MRI is useful for classifying patients as SpA.

3.1 Protocol

An MRI of the sacroiliac joints is conducted with the patient in the supine position. Semicoronal T1w sequence and either a STIR or fat-saturated T2-weighted (T2FS) sequence, should be included in the routine evaluation of the SIJs by MRI. T1w images are mandatory for evaluation of structural (chronic) changes, such as bone erosion, new bone formation and fat infiltrations. Active inflammatory changes are visualized best by fat saturated T2-weighted turbo spin-echo sequence or a short tau inversion recovery (STIR) sequence, which can detect bone marrow edema [20].

Bone marrow abnormalities in both sacroiliac joints and spine are detected almost equally well with the STIR and contrast-enhanced T1w FS sequences in patients with SpA, so contrast injection is generally not needed [21].

The whole sacral bone image should be included both its anterior to its posterior border, which usually requires at least 10–12 slices. Transverse slices are useful for assessment of the posterior parts of the spine. However, for routine imaging of the spine transverse sequences are time consuming and therefore less feasible.

Characteristic lesions in the sacroiliac joints and the spine of patients with AS [8].

ASAS group defines sacroiliitis by MRI as 'active inflammatory lesions of sacroiliac joints with definite bone marrow edema/osteitis' as suggestive of spondyloarthritis [22].

Inflammatory (active) changes	Structural (chronic) changes
Sacroiliitis/bone marrow edema/osteitis	Subchondral sclerosis
Synovitis	Erosions
Capsulitis	Fat metaplasia
Enthesitis	Ankylosis

3.2 Inflammatory (active) changes

3.2.1 Bone marrow edema (BME)

Bone marrow edema is the term given to abnormal fluid signal seen within the bone marrow on MRI and reflects osteitis. BME is hypointense in T1 sequences and hyperintense in T2-FS and STIR sequences. To define it as sacroiliitis, BME should be associated with SIJ (periarticularly located), approximately 1 cm in width (especially in the inferior part of the joint), and should be observed in at least 2 consecutive sequences or more than 1 lesion in a single image. The stronger the signal intensity, the stronger the association with the disease. BME generally associated with structural damage such as erosions or sclerosis (**Figures 3** and **4**).

Bone edema and osteitis are highly suggestive of active sacroiliitis. However, bone edema can be found in other conditions and between 2.6 and 20% in healthy patients [23].

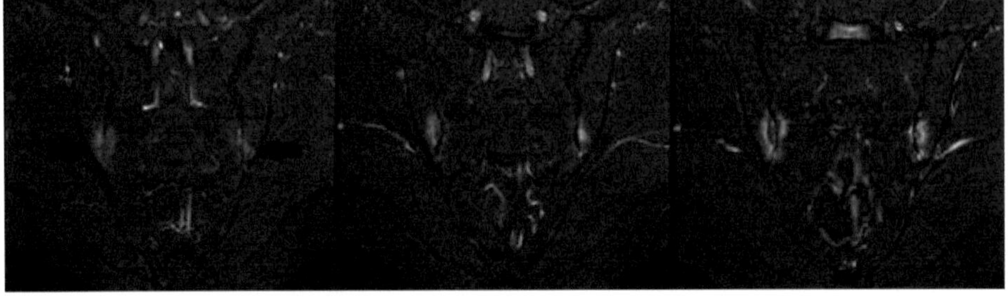

Figure 3.
STIR sequences of sacroiliac joint demonstrates bilateral bone marrow edema on three consecutive slices.

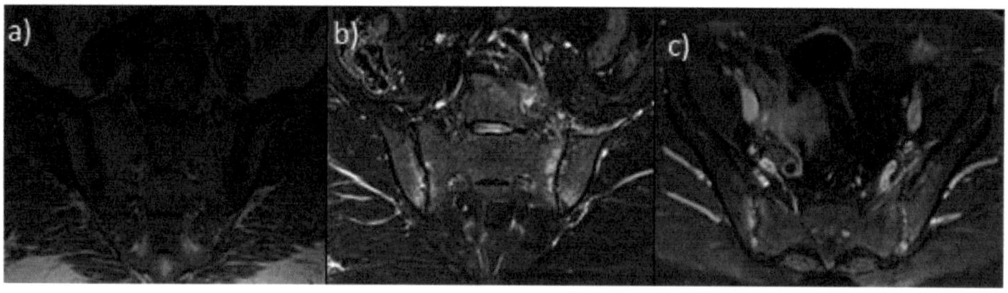

Figure 4.
(a) T1-weighted image shows bilateral large erosions. (b) STIR images demonstrate bilateral bone marrow edema on SIJs. (c) Prominent synovitis is shown with T1-weighted contrast enhanced images.

3.2.2 Synovitis, capsulitis and enthesitis

Synovitis, capsulitis and enthesitis can be demonstrated on contrast-enhanced T1w images. STIR sequences do not differentiate synovitis from joint fluid (**Figure 5**).

3.3 Structural (chronic) changes

3.3.1 Subchondral sclerosis

Sclerosis is seen as low signal intensity areas in all sequences (T1, STIR, T2 FS) and shows no signal enhancement after contrast medium administration. Sclerosis should extend at least 5 mm from the SI joint space.

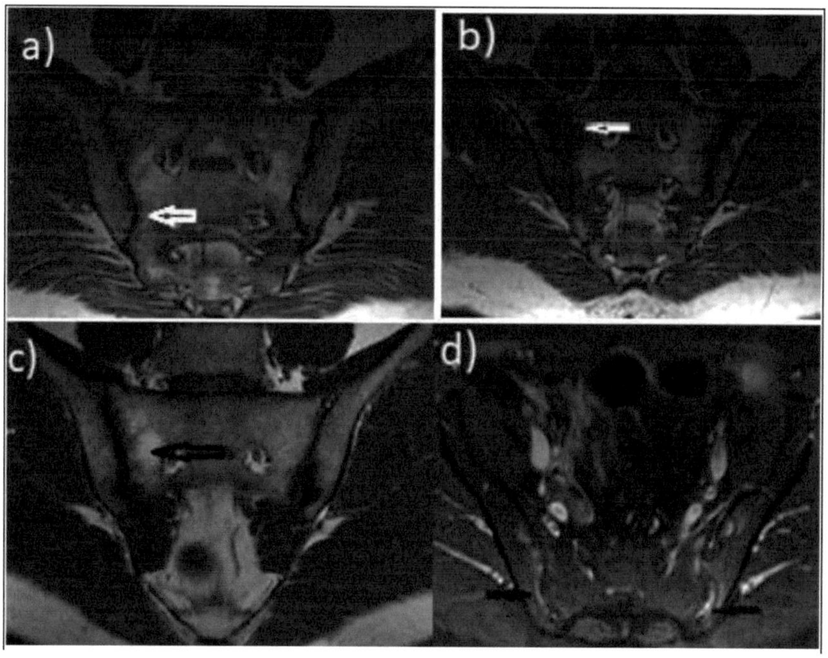

Figure 5.
(a) Right iliac and sacral erosions is seen on T1-weighted image. (b) large subchondral sclerosis (T1-w). (c) subchondral fat metaplasia (T1-w). (d) bilaterally synovitis on T1-w contrast enhanced image.

3.3.2 Erosions

Erosions are bony defects at the joint margin. Erosions may occur throughout the cartilaginous compartment of the joint. Erosions initially appear as single lesions. Confluence of erosions may be seen as pseudodilation of the sacroiliac joints. Erosions are seen as low signal intensity on T1-weighted images. T2 gradient-echo or T1 fat saturated sequences maybe more useful in detecting erosions.

3.3.3 Periarticular fat deposition

Periarticular fat deposition is characterized on MRI by an increased signal intensity on T1-weighted images and low signal intensity on T2w FS and STIR sequences. Accumulation occurs mostly periarticular bone marrow areas and is not a specific finding for AS.

3.3.4 Ankylosis

Ankylosis is bony bridges across the joint with low signal intensity on all MRI sequences.

The presence of synovitis, capsulitis, or enthesitis without concomitant subchondral bone marrow edema/osteitis is not sufficient for making a diagnosis of active sacroiliitis. Structural lesions such as fat deposition, sclerosis, erosions or bony ankylosis represents previous inflammation.

3.4 ASAS positive MRI

ASAS defines sacroiliitis as BME/osteitis in the subchondral bone. There should be BME at least 2 consecutive sequences or more than 1 lesion in a single image [24].

3.5 SPINE

Active lesions of the spine in AS patients are spondylitis, spondylodiscitis and arthritis of the facet, costovertebral and costotransverse joints. Enthesitis may affect the interspinal and supraspinal ligaments and the interosseous ligaments of the sacroiliac joints.

3.5.1 Spondylitis

Spinal MRI shows us active spinal lesions, disease activity and response to therapy. Inflammation of vertebral body can be seen as shiny corners, Romanus lesions and vertebral osteitis, most frequently seen in the thoracolumbar region (T10-T12). The typical appearance of spondylitis is not limited to vertebral edges but also spread to the entire vertebral body. Syndesmophytes occur as a result of inflammation and repair reaction (**Figure 6**) [25, 26].

3.5.2 Spondylodiscitis

Spinal inflammation also seen in the intervertebral space (diskitis) and diskitis with vertebral body inflammation (spondylodiskitis-Andersson lesions). Andersson lesion is inflammation involving the intervertebral disc and adjacent vertebrae. Asymptomatic spondylodiskitis may occur in early disease [27].

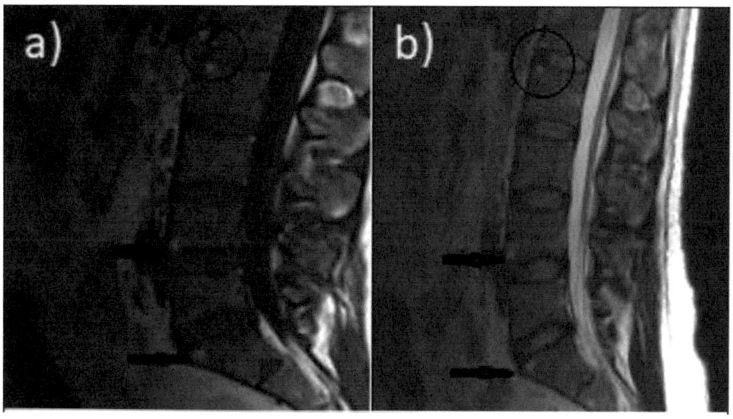

Figure 6.
Sagittal MRI view of lumbar spine in AS patient. (a) T1-w image and (b) T2-w FS images demonstrate vertebral endplate osteitis (Romanus lesions).

3.6 Scoring the MRI

Several systems for assessment of disease activity in the sacroiliac joints and in the spine have been proposed. The SPARCC method had the highest sensitivity to change [28].

3.6.1 SPARCC

This method is based on the evaluation on STIR sequence six consecutive semi-coronal slices focusing on the synovial part of the SIJ. Six coronal slices are assessed and only STIR sequences are scored. The sacroiliac joint is divided into four quadrants (upper iliac, lower iliac, upper sacral and lower sacral) and each quadrant is examined

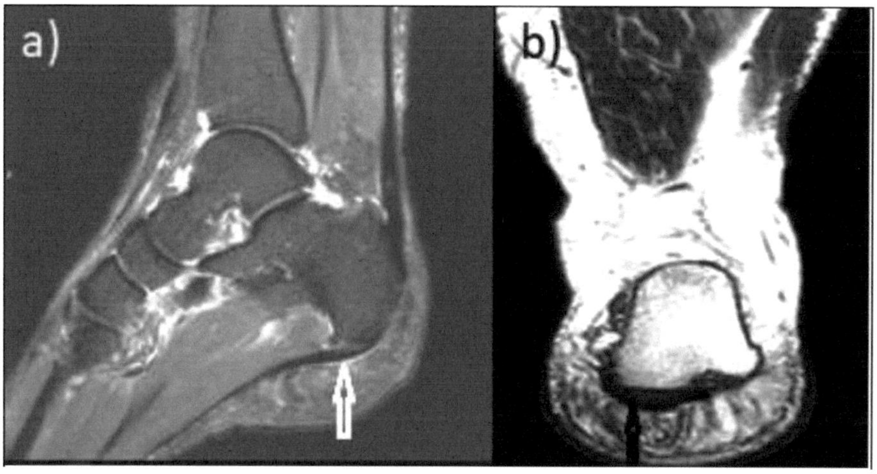

Figure 7.
AS patients also have peripheral clinical findings as arthritis and enthesitis. (a) sagittal image shows tibiotalar-talonavicular arthritis with plantar fasciitis (white arrow). (b) T1-w axial image also demonstrates plantar fasciitis (black arrow).

separately. For each quadrant, it is recorded whether it has an hyperintense lesion in the STIR sequence. Each quadrant is also scored due to its signal intensity. Total maximum score is 72 [29]. Assessment of the chronic inflammatory changes is important for disease monitoring.

MRI also help us to determine peripheral lesions of AS, like peripheral arthritis and enthesitis. Achilles tendon and plantar fascia are the most affected sites of entesitis (**Figure 7**).

4. Computed tomography

CT permits imaging the structural changes without superimposition of overlying structures. CT shows chronic changes more clearly than conventional radiography.

Semicoronal CT is used for the diagnosis of sacroiliitis. Semicoronal technique permits an overview of the cartilaginous and ligamentous portions of the SIJ with less radiation dose—6–8 contiguous 5-mm slices [30].

CT can detect osteoporosis or osteosclerosis quite well but these changes are very nonspecific. The primary value of CT in AS is its ability to detect and clearly define erosion of bone at any joint or enthesis, and for documenting fractures.

Typical changes for sacroiliitis at CT are joint erosions, subchondral sclerosis and ankylosis [31]. Joint space narrowing and pseudo-widening can be viewed clearly (**Figure 8**). However, CT findings may be misleading in elderly patients because subchondral sclerosis in the iliac part of the SIJs can be seen due to aging.

CT is superior to MRI, especially in detecting sclerosis, bone production, and chronic bone changes in the ligamentous portion of the joint. But CT cannot reveal bone marrow edema, which makes the diagnosis of active sacroiliitis. A new promising technique; low-dose CT of the SIJs may replace CR as a method of structural damage and new bone formation monitoring [32, 33].

In the spine, CT can demonstrate complications of the disease such as spondylodiscitis or spinal fracture.

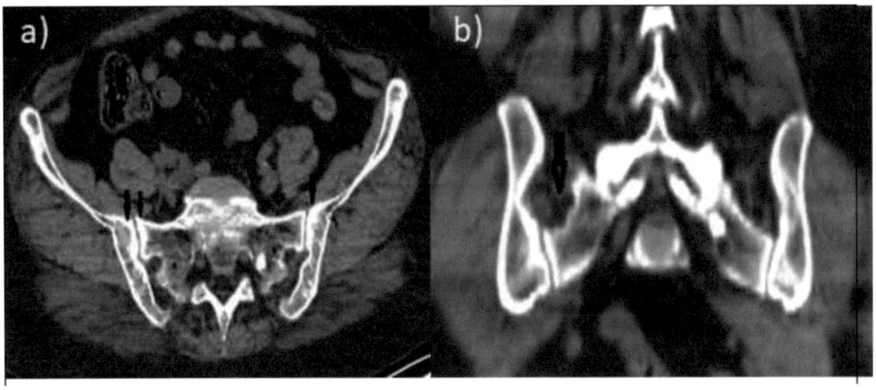

Figure 8.
CT images of sacroiliac joints (a) axial CT image demonstrates bilateral subchondral sclerosis (b) coronal image shows right sided large erosions.

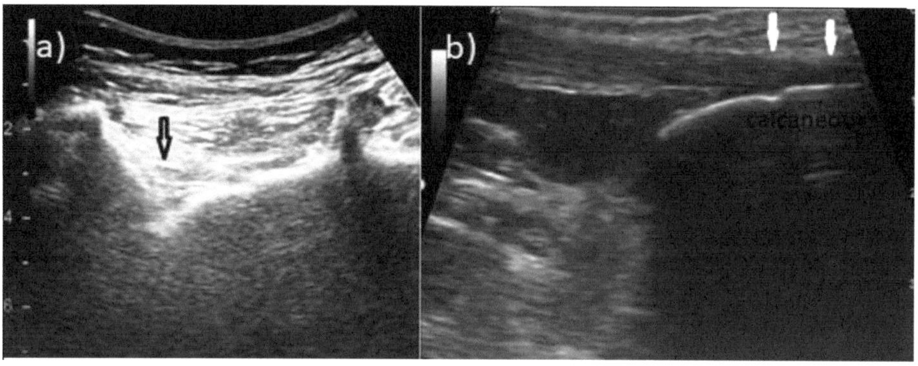

Figure 9.
(a) Normal view of sacroiliac joint (b) normal US view of Achilles tendon.

5. Ultrasonography

Ultrasonography (US) is an evolving imaging technique increasingly used by the rheumatologist in daily clinical practice. The role of US in assessment of sacroiliac and spine involvement in AS and other types of axial SpA is minimal [34]. Only the superficial part of the SIJs is accessible to visualization by US including the surrounding soft tissue structures and the posterior stabilizing ligaments, while the cartilaginous portion is inaccessible by this imaging modality.

However, US can be used to guide SIJ corticosteroid injections, particularly where these appear to be the primary affected joints [35–38].

Ultrasonography is more useful in the diagnosis of peripheral involvement of the disease. US has a high sensitivity and specificity in the diagnosis of Achilles and plantar enthesitis, especially using the power Doppler. It is also a guide for interventional treatment for arthritis and enthesitis (**Figure 9**).

While US assessment is safe, noninvasive, comparably cheap and conveys no radiation, it is highly operator-dependent and influenced by the quality of the US equipment.

6. Radionuclide methods

6.1 Bone scintigraphy with technetium-99 labeled methylene diphosphate

Bone scintigraphy can be used to detect inflammation by demonstrating increased uptake in the sacroiliac joints [39]. It also gives the chance to evaluate the inflammation quantitatively by comparing the radionuclide signal intensity [39, 40]. But it has a limited value in detecting AS in clinical practice. Scintigraphy of sacroiliac joints has low sensitivity for diagnosis of suspected or established ankylosing spondylitis.

A review by Song et al. on the performance of bone scintigraphy showed an overall sensitivity of about 50% and specificity not higher than about 80% for the diagnosis of sacroiliitis [41]. Also, the radiation exposure of bone scintigraphy limits its daily use in patients with suspected AS.

6.2 Single-photon emission computed tomography (SPECT) and combined SPECT-CT

Quality and sensitivity of the bone scintigraphy can be increased with using SPECT. SPECT provides a better anatomical evaluation of the joint. SPECT has been shown to be superior in quantifying the SIJ to sacrum ratio [42]. Kim et al. showed that SPECT with low dose CT is superior to bone scintigraphy in demonstrating early sacroiliitis, with sensitivity of 80% and specificity of 84% [43].

7. Novel/future modalities

7.1 Whole-body MRI (wbMRI)

In recent years, new magnetic resonance imaging modalities has been developed for diagnosing AS patients. Multichannel systems and multiple coils are used to scan larger areas, like wbMRI. This MRI modality allows a clearer assessment of peripheral involvement [44, 45]. wbMRI includes T1w and STIR sequences of the entire spine, shoulder girdle, arms, anterior chest wall, pelvis including the SIJs and the lower extremities [46]. wbMRI reduces imaging times and spatial resolution is similar to standard MRI [46].

This modality is mostly helpful for the assessment of enthesitis [47, 48]. wbMRI may contribute for the early diagnosis of AS and was shown to detect active inflammation and structural changes in active nr-axSpA and AS [45, 49].

7.2 Diffusion-weighted MRI (DWI)

a new MRI modality, the image contrast is yielded by the random motion of the water molecules in different biological tissue environments, within the cellular and extracellular tissue compartments, providing both quantitative [apparent diffusion coefficient (ADC)] and qualitative functional information [50]. Inflammation leads to higher ADC values through increased water in extracellular spaces. DWI was shown to identify active sacroiliitis based on conventional MRI on qualitative analysis, and to differentiate active from inactive sacroiliitis by quantitative ADC measurements [51]. Preliminary data with high-resolution MRI show an increased detection rate of erosions on the SIJs when compared to conventional MRI and low-dose CT [52].

8. Differential diagnosis

BME of the SIJ can be observed in several conditions other than AS. Most common conditions are infectious sacroiliitis, osteitis condensans ilii, diffuse idiopathic skeletal hyperostosis (DISH), and pelvic fractures.

BME/osteitis in infectious sacroiliitis extends to the surrounding soft tissue [53]. MRI detects early signs of infection, while CR is usually normal in the first few weeks.

8.1 Osteitis condensans ilii

Osteitis condensans ilii is depicted as a triangular-shaped area of sclerosis of the iliac side of the SIJ, on MRI as on CR or CT [54]. It is frequently seen in middle-aged women after pregnancy, although it can rarely occur in men (**Figure 10**).

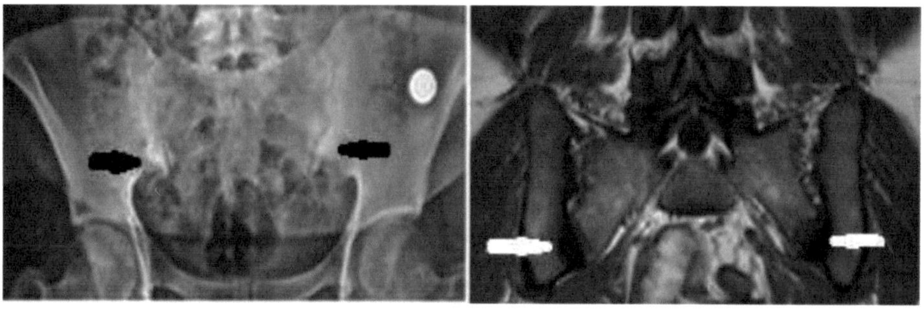

Figure 10.
Osteitis condensans ilii. Both conventional radiography and MRI (STIR) demonstrates bilateral inferior triangular shaped sclerosis.

8.2 DISH

DISH is characterized by wide, bulky osteophytes with concomitant ossification of the anterior longitudinal ligament. The ossification extends three to four consecutive vertebrae and osteophytes can be seen at the shoulder, elbow, knee, or calcaneus [55]. The absence of ankylosis at the facet-joint interface and absence of sacroiliac joint erosion, sclerosis, or fusion are used in the distinction of DISH and AS (**Figure 11**) [56].

8.3 Insufficiency fractures

Insufficiency fractures of the sacrum may present with low back pain and as the fracture line is not always visible, may lead to a misdiagnosis. MR image may be confused with bone marrow edema (**Figure 12**).

8.4 CPPD

Calcium pyrophospahtel deposition in the spine can cause spine stiffness with bony ankylosis and can be misdiagnosed with AS or DISH. In addition, crystal

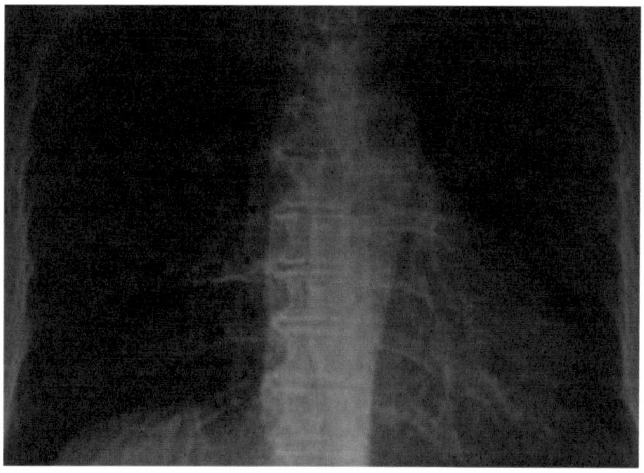

Figure 11.
AP view thoracal spine shows right sided large osteophytes on the anterior longitudinal ligament in patient with DISH.

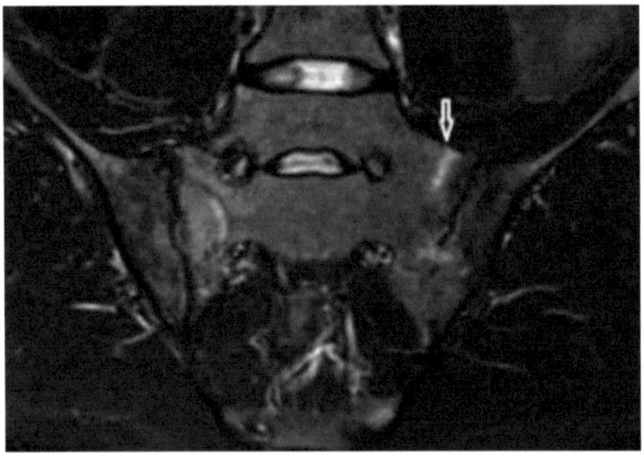

Figure 12.
STIR image of sacroiliac joint in AS patient also shows insufficiency fracture in left superior sacral bone.

deposition may lead to spinal cord compression syndromes. CPPD should be in the differential diagnosis of AS especially in elderly and patients with familial chondrocalcinosis.

8.5 Postpartum transient sacroilitis

Inflammatory low back pain can be seen in young women in the postpartum period and bone marrow edema can be seen in MR imaging. Transient sacroiliitis should not be confused with AS so MRI is not recommended in the first year of delivery to screen AS (**Figure 13**).

The most important differential diagnoses in the spine are degenerative/ mechanical lesions, blood vessels and hemangioma, fractures, and septic spondylitis/ spondylodiscitis.

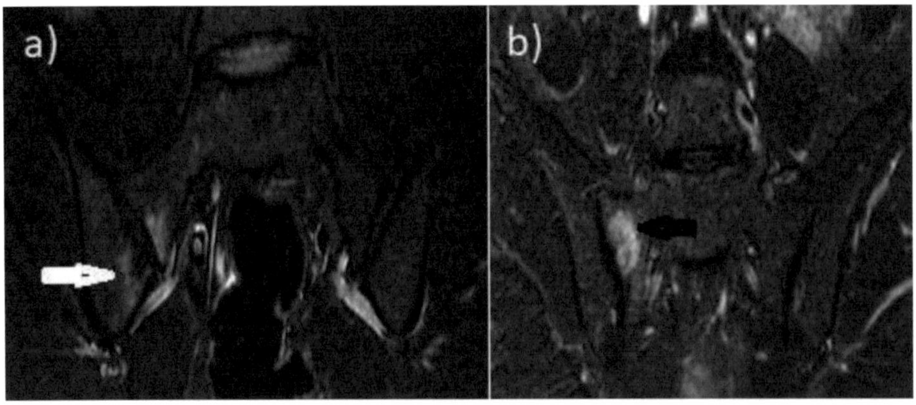

Figure 13.
(a) 26 year old male patient having inflammatory back pain after using isotretinoin and T2 FS image shows bone marrow edema on inferior right SIJ. (b) 28 year old female with inflammatory back pain 4 months after delivery. STIR sequence demonstrates bone marrow edema on the right superior sacral side of the joint, favoring postpartum transient sacroiliitis.

9. Recommendations for imaging

The diagnosis of AS is delayed approximately 7 years in many patients [57, 58]. The main reason for the delay in diagnosis is that radiographic sacroiliitis must be present in the x-ray for diagnosis among the modified New York criteria. These criteria are quite specific in patients with established disease, but they are insensitive for diagnosing early stages of disease. MRI is mostly preferred to prevent delay in diagnosis and to detect early signs of inflammation. Despite all the developments and different techniques in the field of imaging in recent years, conventional radiography is still the gold standard imaging method, especially for the assessment of structural damage.

Compared to other imaging modalities (conventional radiography, CT, scintigraphy), MRI is significantly superior in both detecting disease and showing active lesions [59, 60].

9.1 EULAR recommendations for diagnosis of axial SpA

In 2015, European League Against Rheumatism (EULAR) taskforce developed recommendations on the use of musculoskeletal imaging in the clinical management of axial Spondyloarthritis [61]. Conventional radiography is the first recommended imaging method. In young patients with short symptom duration, MRI can be preferred in the first line imaging. MRI of the spine is not generally recommended to diagnose axial SpA. Imaging modalities, other than conventional radiography and MRI are generally not recommended in the diagnosis of axial SpA. Monitoring disease activity MRI with STIR sequences are sufficient to detect inflammation. Conventional radiography of the SI joints and/or spine are used to monitor structural changes.

Conflict of interest

The author declare no conflict of interest.

Abbreviations

ADC	apparent diffusion coefficient
AP	anteroposterior
AS	ankylosing spondylitis
ASAS	assessment of spondyloArthritis international society
axSpA	axial spondyloarthritis
BASRI	bath ankylosing spondylitis radiology index
BME	bone marrow edema
CR	conventional radiography
CT	computed tomography
DISH	diffuse idiopathic skeletal hyperostosis
DWI	diffusion-weighted MRI
EULAR	European league against rheumatism
MRI	magnetic resonance imaging
mSASSS	modified stoke ankylosing spondylitis spinal score
nr-axSpA	nonradiographic axial spondyloarthritis

SIJ	sacroiliac joint
SPARCC	spondyloarthritis research consortium of Canada
SPECT	single-photon emission computerized tomography
STIR	short tau inversion recovery
T1-W	T1 weighted
T2 FS	T2 fat saturated
US	ultrasonography
wbMRI	whole-body MRI

Author details

Esra Dilsat Bayrak
Department of Rheumatology, Acıbadem University Acıbadem Atakent Hospital, İstanbul, Turkey

*Address all correspondence to: drdilsat@hotmail.com

References

[1] Braun J, Sieper J. Ankylosing spondylitis. Lancet. 2007;**369**:1379-1390. DOI: 10.1016/S0140-6736(07)60635-7

[2] Puhakkas KB, Melsen F, Jurik AG, et al. MR imaging of the normal sacroiliac joint with correlation to histology. Skeletal Radiology. 2004;**33**:15-28

[3] Prassopoulos PK, Faflia CP, Voloudaki AE, Gourtsoyiannis NC. Sacroiliac joints: Anatomical variants on CT. Journal of Computer Assisted Tomography. 1999;**23**(2):323-327. DOI: 10.1097/00004728-199903000-00029 PMID: 10096348

[4] Guglielmi G, Scalzo G, Cascavilla A, Carotti M, Salaffi F, Grassi W. Imaging of the sacroiliac joint involvement in seronegative spondylarthropathies. Clinical Rheumatology. 2009;**28**:1007-1019. DOI: 10.1007/s10067-009-1192-1

[5] Lampignano J, Kendrick LE. Bontrager's Textbook of Radiographic Positioning and Related Anatomy. 2017:279-280. ISBN: 9780323399661

[6] van der Linden S, Valkenburg HA, Cats A. Evaluation of diagnostic criteria for ankylosing spondylitis. A proposal for modification of the New York criteria. Arthritis and Rheumatism. 1984;**27**:361-368

[7] Rudwaleit M, van der Heijde D, Landewé R, Listing J, Akkoc N, Brandt J, et al. The development of assessment of spondyloarthritis international society classification criteria for axial spondyloarthritis (part II): Validation and final selection. Annals of the Rheumatic Diseases. 2009;**68**:777-783. DOI: 10.1136/ard.2009.108233

[8] Poddubnyy D, Brandt H, Vahldiek J, et al. The frequency of non-radiographic axial spondyloarthritis in relation to symptom duration in patients referred because of chronic back pain: Results from the Berlin early spondyloarthritis clinic. Annals of the Rheumatic Diseases. 2012;**71**:1998-2001

[9] Sieper J et al. Progression of radiographic damage in patients with ankylosing spondylitis: Defining the central role of syndesmophytes. Annals of the Rheumatic Diseases. 2007;**66**:910-915. DOI: 10.1136/ard.2006.066415

[10] Braun J, van der Heijde D. Imaging and scoring in ankylosing spondylitis. Best Practice & Research. Clinical Rheumatology. 2002;**16**:573-604. DOI: 10.1053/berh.2002.0250

[11] Baraliakos X, Listing J, Rudwaleit M, Haibel H, Brandt J, Sieper J, et al. Progression of radiographic damage in patients with ankylosing spondylitis: Defining the central role of syndesmophytes. Annals of Rheumatic Diseases. 2007;**66**(7):910-915. DOI: 10.1136/ard.2006.066415. Epub February 28, 2007

[12] Ostergaard M, Lambert RG. Imaging in ankylosing spondylitis. Therapeutic Advances in Musculoskeletal Disease. 2012;**4**(4):301-311. DOI: 10.1177/1759720X11436240 PMID: 22859929; PMCID: PMC3403247

[13] Ramiro S, van Tubergen A, van der Heijde D, Stolwijk C, Bookelman G, Dougados M, et al. Brief report: Erosions and sclerosis on radiographs precede the subsequent development of syndesmophytes at the same site: A twelve-year prospective followup of patients with ankylosing spondylitis. Arthritis & Rhematology. 2014;**66**(10):2773-2779. DOI: 10.1002/art.38775

[14] Creemers MC, Franssen MJ, van't Hof MA, Gribnau FW, van de Putte LB, van Riel PL. Assessment of outcome in ankylosing spondylitis: An extended radiographic scoring system. Annals of Rheumatic Disorder. 2005;**64**(1):127-129. DOI: 10.1136/ard.2004.020503 Epub March 29, 2004

[15] MacKay K, Mack C, Brophy S, Calin A. The bath ankylosing spondylitis radiology index (BASRI): A new, validated approach to disease assessment. Arthritis and Rheumatism. 1998;**41**:2263-2270. DOI: 10.1002/1529-0131(199812)41:12<2263:AID-ART23>3.0.CO;2-I

[16] Mackay K, Brophy S, Mack C, Doran M, Calin A. The development and validation of a radiographic grading system for the hip in ankylosing spondylitis: The bath ankylosing spondylitis radiology hip index. J Rheumatol. 2000;**27**:2866-2872

[17] Wanders AJ, Landewé RB, Spoorenberg A, et al. What is the most appropriate radiologic scoring method for ankylosing spondylitis? A comparison of the available methods based on the outcome measures in rheumatology clinical trials filter. Arthritis and Rheumatism. 2004;**50**:2622-2632

[18] Creemers MC, Franssen MJ, van'tHof MA, Gribnau FW, van de Putte LB, van Riel PL. Assessment of outcome in ankylosing spondylitis: An extended radiographic scoring system. Annals of the Rheumatic Diseases. 2005;**64**:127-129

[19] Weber U, Lambert RGW, Pedersen SJ, Hodler J, Østergaard M, Maksymowych WP. Assessment of structural lesions in sacroiliac joints enhances diagnostic utility of magnetic resonance imaging in early spondylarthritis. Arthritis Care Res (Hoboken). 2010;**62**:1763-1771. DOI: 10.1002/acr.20312

[20] Braun J, van der Heijde D. Imaging and scoring in ankylosing spondylitis. Best Practice & Research. Clinical Rheumatology. 2002;**4**:573-604 PMID: 12406428

[21] Baraliakos X, Hermann KG, Landewe R, Listing J, Golder W, Brandt J, et al. Assessment of acute spinal inflammation in patients with ankylosing spondylitis by magnetic resonance imaging: A comparison between contrast enhanced T1 and short tau inversion recovery (STIR) sequences. Annals of the Rheumatic Diseases. 2005;**64**:1141-1144

[22] Sieper J, Rudwaleit M, Baraliakos X, et al. The Assessment of Spondylo Arthritis international Society (ASAS) handbook: A guide to assess spondyloarthritis. Annals of Rheumatic Diseases. 2009;**68**:ii1-ii44

[23] Weber U, Pedersen SJ, Østergaard M, Rufibach K, Lambert RG, Maksymowych WP, et al. Can erosions on MRI of the sacroiliac joints be reliably detected in patients with ankylosing spondylitis? A cross-sectional study. Arthritis Research & Therapy. 2012;**14**:R124

[24] Rudwaleit M, Jurik AG, Hermann KG, Landewé R, van der Heijde D, Baraliakos X, et al. Defining active sacroiliitis on magnetic resonance imaging (MRI) for classification of axial spondyloarthritis: A consensual approach by the ASAS/OMERACT MRI group. Annals of the Rheumatic Diseases. 2009;**68**:1520-1527. DOI: 10.1136/ard.2009.110767

[25] Baraliakos X, Herman KG, Landewe R, et al. Assessment of acute spinal inflammation in patients with ankylosing spondylitis by magnetic

resonance imaging (MRI): A comparison between contrast enhanced T1 and short-tau inversion recovery (STIR) sequences. Annals of the Rheumatic Diseases. 2005;**64**(8):1141-1144

[26] Braun J, Baraliakos X, Golder W, et al. Analysing chronic spinal changes in ankylosing spondylitis: A systematic comparison of conventional x-rays with magnetic resonance imaging using established and new scoring systems. Annals of the Rheumatic Diseases. 2004;**63**(9):1046-1055

[27] Wienads K, Lukas P, Albrecht HJ. Clinical value of MR tomography of spondylodiskitis in ankylosing spondylitis. The Journal of Rheumatology. 1990;**49**(6):356-360

[28] Lukas C, Braun J, van der Heijde D, Hermann KG, Rudwaleit M, Østergaard M, et al. Scoring inflammatory activity of the spine by magnetic resonance imaging in ankylosing spondylitis: A multireader experiment. The Journal of Rheumatology. 2007;**34**:862-870

[29] Maksymowych WP, Inman RD, Salonen D, Dhillon SS, Williams M, Stone M, et al. Spondyloarthritis research consortium of Canada magnetic resonance imaging index for assessment of sacroiliac joint inflammation in ankylosing spondylitis. Arthritis and Rheumatism. 2005;**53**:703-709. DOI: 10.1002/art.21445

[30] Carrera GF, Foley WD, Kozin F, Ryan L, Lawson TL. CT of sacroiliitis. AJR. American Journal of Roentgenology. 1981;**136**:41-46. DOI: 10.2214/ajr.136.1.41

[31] Taggart AJ, Desai SM, Iveson JM, Verow PW. Computerized tomography of the sacro-iliac joints in the diagnosis of sacro-iliitis. British Journal of Rheumatology. 1984;**23**:258-266. DOI: 10.1093/rheumatology/23.4.258

[32] Gao D, Li KP, Wen QF, Zhu J, Zhang JL, Huang F. A preliminary exploration of low-dose semicoronal CT of the sacroiliac joints in the diagnosis of ankylosing spondylitis. Zhonghua Nei Ke Za Zhi. 2016;**55**:355-360. DOI: 10.3760/cma.j.i ssn.0578-1426.2016.05.005

[33] Maksymowych WP, Lambert RG. Spondyloarthritis: Lowdose CT for spondyloarthritis—A brilliant new chapter? Nature Reviews Rheumatology. 2018;**14**:130-131. DOI: 10.1038/nrrheum.2018.4

[34] Klauser A, Halpern EJ, Frauscher F, Gvozdic D, Duftner C, Springer P, et al. Inflammatory low back pain: High negative predictive value of contrast-enhanced color Doppler ultrasound in the detection of inflamed sacroiliac joints. Arthritis and Rheumatism. 2005;**53**:440-444

[35] Pekkafahli MZ, Kiralp MZ, Başekim CC, Silit E, Mutlu H, Oztürk E, et al. Sacroiliac joint injections performed with sonographic guidance. Journal of Ultrasound in Medicine. 2003;**22**:553-559. DOI. 10.7863/jum.2003.22.6.553

[36] Klauser A, De Zordo T, Feuchtner G, Sögner P, Schirmer M, Gruber J, et al. Feasibility of ultrasound-guided sacroiliac joint injection consideringsonoanatomic landmarks at two different levels in cadavers and patients. Arthritis Care and Research. 2008;**59**:1618-1624. DOI: 10.1002/art.24204

[37] Chang W-H, Lew HL, Chen CPC. Ultrasound-guided sacroiliac joint injection technique. American Journal of Physical Medicine & Rehabilitation. 2013;**92**:278-279. DOI: 10.1097/PHM.0b013e318278d108

[38] Perry JM, Colberg RE, Dault SL, Beason DP, Tresgallo RA. A cadaveric study assessing the accuracy of

ultrasound-guided sacroiliac joint injections. Polymyalgia Rheumatica. 2016;**8**:1168-1172. DOI: 10.1016/j.pmrj.2016.05.002

[39] Akdeniz O, Alayli G, Tosun FC, Diren B, Cengiz K, Selüuk MB, et al. Early spondyloarthropathy: Scintigraphic, biological, and clinical findings in MRI-positive patients. Clinical Rheumatology. 2008;**27**:469-474. DOI: 10.1007/s10067-007-0730-y

[40] Koç ZP, Cengiz AK, Aydın F, Samancı N, Yazısız V, Koca SS, et al. Sacroiliac indicis increase the specificity of bone scintigraphy in the diagnosis of sacroiliitis. Molecular Imaging and Radionuclide Therapy. 2015;**24**:8-14. DOI: 10.4274/mirt.40427

[41] Song IH, Carrasco-Fernández J, Rudwaleit M, Sieper J. The diagnostic value of scintigraphy in assessing sacroiliitis in ankylosing spondylitis: A systematic literature research. Annals of the Rheumatic Diseases. 2008;**67**:1535-1540. DOI: 10.1136/ard.2007.083089

[42] Jacobsson H, Larsson SA, Vesterskold L, Lindvall N. The application of single photon emission computed tomography to the diagnosis of ankylosing spondylitis of the spine. The British Journal of Radiology. 1984;**57**:133-140. DOI: 10.1259/0007-1285-57-674-133

[43] Kim Y, Suh M, Kim YK, Lee H-Y, Shin K. The usefulness of bone SPECT/CT imaging with volume of interest analysis in early axial spondyloarthritis. BMC Musculoskeletal Disorders. 2015;**16**:9. DOI: 10.1186/s12891-015-0465-x

[44] Weber U, Pfirrmann CWA, Kissling RO, Hodler J, Zanetti M. Whole body MR imaging in ankylosing spondylitis: A descriptive pilot study in patients with suspected early and active confirmed ankylosing spondylitis. BMC Musculoskeletal Disorders. 2007;**8**:20. DOI: 10.1186/1471-2474-8-20

[45] Mager AK, Althoff CE, Sieper J, Hamm B, Hermann KG. Role of wholebody magnetic resonance imaging in diagnosing early spondyloarthritis. European Journal of Radiology. 2009;**71**:182-188. DOI: 10.1016/j.ejrad.2009.04.051

[46] Baraliakos X, Landewé R, Hermann KG, Listing J, Golder W, Brandt J, et al. Inflammation in ankylosing spondylitis: A systematic description of the extent and frequency of acute spinal changes using magnetic resonance imaging. Annals of the Rheumatic Diseases. 2005;**64**:730-734

[47] Poggenborg RP, Eshed I, Østergaard M, Sørensen IJ, Møller JM, Madsen OR, et al. Enthesitis in patients with psoriatic arthritis, axial spondyloarthritis and healthy subjects assessed by "head-to-toe" whole-body MRI and clinical examination. Annals of the Rheumatic Diseases. 2015;**74**:823-829. DOI: 10.1136/annrheumdis-2013-204239

[48] Poggenborg RP, Pedersen SJ, Eshed I, Sørensen IJ, Møller JM, Madsen OR, et al. Head-to-toe whole-body MRI in psoriatic arthritis, axial spondyloarthritis and healthy subjects: First steps towards global inflammation and damage scores of peripheral and axial joints. Rheumatology (Oxford). 2015;**54**:1039-1049. DOI: 10.1093/rheumatology/keu439

[49] Althoff CE, Sieper J, Song I-H, Haibel H, Weiß A, Diekhoff T, et al. Active inflammation and structural change in early active axial spondyloarthritis as detected by whole-body MRI. Annals of the Rheumatic Diseases. 2013;**72**:967-973. DOI: 10.1136/annrheumdis-2012-201545

[50] Raya JG, Dietrich O, Reiser MF, Baur-Melnyk A. Methods and applications of diffusion imaging of vertebral bone marrow. Journal of Magnetic Resonance Imaging. 2006;**24**:1207-1220. DOI: 10.1002/jmri.20748

[51] Gašperšič N, Serša I, Jevtič V, Tomšič M, Praprotnik S. Monitoring ankylosing spondylitis therapy by dynamic contrast-enhanced and diffusion-weighted magnetic resonance imaging. Skeletal Radiology. 2008;**37**:123-131. DOI: 10.1007/s00256-007-0407-2

[52] Diekhoff T, Greese J, Krohn M, Huppertz A, Hamm B, Hermann KG. OP0050 erosion detection on the Si-Joints – a comparison between X-Ray, low dose CT and MRI including high resolution sequences. Annals of the Rheumatic Diseases. 2014;**73**:79-80. DOI: 10.1136/annrheumdis-2014-eular.2145

[53] Stürzenbecher A, Braun J, Paris S, Biedermann T, Hamm B, Bollow M. MR imaging of septic sacroiliitis. Skeletal Radiology. 2000;**29**:439-446. DOI: 10.1007/s002560000242

[54] Mitra R. Osteitis condensans ilii. Rheumatology International. 2010;**30**:293-296. DOI: 10.1007/s00296-009-1100-7

[55] Belanger TA, Rowe DE. Diffuse idiopathic skeletal hyperostosis: Musculoskeletal manifestations. The Journal of the American Academy of Orthopaedic Surgeons. 2001;**9**(4):258-267 [PubMed]

[56] Arad U, Elkayam O, Eshed I. Magnetic resonance imaging in diffuse idiopathic skeletal hyperostosis: Similarities to axial spondyloarthritis. Clinical Rheumatology. 2017;**36**:1545-1549. DOI: 10.1007/s10067-017-3617-6

[57] Zink A, Braun J, Listing J, Wollenhaupt J. Disability and handicap in rheumatoid arthritis and ankylosing spondylitis—Results from the German rheumatological database. German Collaborative Arthritis Centers. Journal of Rheumatology. 2000;**27**:613-622

[58] Feldtkeller E. Age at disease onset and delayed diagnosis of spondyloarthropathies. Zeitschrift für Rheumatologie. 1999;**58**:21-30

[59] Battafarano DF, West SG, Rak KM, Fortenbery EJ, Chantelois AE. Comparison of bone scan, computed tomography, and magnetic resonance imaging in the diagnosis of active sacroiliitis. Seminars in Arthritis and Rheumatism. 1993;**23**(3):161-176, ISSN: 0049-0172. DOI: 10.1016/S0049-0172(05)80037-X

[60] Blum U, Buitrago-Tellez C, Mundinger A, Krause T, Laubenberger J, Vaith P, et al. Magnetic resonance imaging (MRI) for detection of active sacroiliitis–a prospective study comparing conventional radiography, scintigraphy, and contrast enhanced MRI. The Journal of Rheumatology 1996;23(12):2107-2115. PMID: 8970049

[61] Mandl P, Navarro-Compán V, Terslev L, et al. EULAR recommendations for the use of imaging in the diagnosis and management of spondyloarthritis in clinical practice. Annals of the Rheumatic Diseases. 2015;**74**:1327-1339

Section 2

Pathogenesis and Treatment of Ankylosing Spondylitis

Chapter 4

Ankylosing Spondylitis Pathogenesis and Pathophysiology

Malini Alexander

Abstract

The pathogenesis and pathophysiology of Ankylosing Spondylitis (AS) is complex and remains only partially understood. Contributory genes including a variety of HLA-B27 subset genes and many other non-HLA genes are implicated in the literature. Novel genes and gene–gene interactions being a continuously evolving area of AS research. Dysregulation of the enteric microbiome with a corresponding aberrant immunological response is recognised in research. Certain infectious agents are thought to play a role. A variety of other influences including environmental exposures, dietary and lifestyle factors and sex hormones appear to play a role in AS pathogenesis. There is emerging evidence that that pathophysiological response in AS is an elaborate combination of both autoinflammatory and autoimmune components, however the IL-17/IL-23 pathway remains the major pathway in AS according to studies to date. The specific mechanisms that lead to characteristic clinical features of AS including sacroiliitis, spondylitis, ankylosis, uveitis and other extra articular manifestations remain occult. Further research to establish these is ongoing.

Keywords: ankylosing spondylitis, HLA-B27, pathogenesis, pathophysiology, seronegative spondyloarthropathy, microbiome dysregulation in spondylitis

1. Introduction

The pathogenesis and pathophysiology of ankylosing spondylitis (AS) involves an extremely complex interplay of factors that can be broadly categorised according to the following key areas:

- Genetic predisposition
- Environmental factors
- Altered gut microbiome and infective triggers
- Enteric wall dysfunction and altered mucosal immunity
- Aberrant systemic immune response and subsequent dysregulation

- Factors associated with the axial skeleton and its entheses
- Factors associated with peripheral entheses and joints
- Aberrations in bone metabolism

This chapter will discuss the major components that contribute to AS pathogenesis. Theories and emerging evidence in the literature are reviewed. Whilst the discussion is divided into various topics for clarity and ease of reading, in reality the factors involved interact in a elaborate matrix of multidirectional feedback all contributing to the ultimate manifestation of AS.

This chapter will review genetic associations with AS. In addition to HLA-B27, there are many novel genes thought to contribute to AS pathogenesis reported in the literature. Section 3.1 reveals the proposed theories of how HLA-B27 specifically leads to an altered immunological response resulting in inflammation.

Autoimmune vs. autoinflammatory immunological features involved in AS pathogenesis and the interplay between disturbancs of the gut microbiome, including by infection and diet leading to altered immune response. The IL-17-23 and IL-12 pathways are discussed in some details.

2. Pathogenesis

2.1 Genetic factors

2.1.1 HLAB27

Human Major Histocompatibility Complex (MHC) class I is also known as Human Leukocyte Antigen (HLA) and is one of the many surface proteins present on all nucleated cells and platelets in the human body [1]. MHC I plays a role in antigen presentation to cytotoxic T cells via the T Cell Receptor (TCR) [1].

Genetic factors contributing to development of AS have been recognised since 1961 leading to the discovery of the HLAB27 gene in 1973 [2]. There is significantly higher concordance between monozygous twins and dizygous twins with AS rates of 63% and 23–27% respectively [2, 3]. Over the years many genes have been identified as associated with AS, however the full picture of gene–gene interactions is yet to be explained.

HLA B27 belongs to the MCH class I receptor family. See the schematic representation in **Figure 1**.

There are 4 domains of this molecule as depicted in **Figure 1**. Regions α1 and α2 are located at the top of the protein where antigen binding occurs (**Figure 2**). The α3 heavy chain is located adjacent to the cell surface partially penetrates the cell membrane. The 4th domain is the β2 microglobulin which is covalently associated with the rest of the HLA B27 molecule [6].

Three main features distinguish HLA B27 from most other HLA class I molecules. Glutanine is substituted for methanine located at the 45 position. The second feature is an unpaired cysteine (Cys67) [7]. This feature enables formation of homodimers and oligomers of free heavy chains which are thought to contribute to development of AS [7] and is discussed in more detail later on in this chapter. Thirdly there is a Lys residue at position 70 that increases reactivity of the cysteine at position 67 [7].

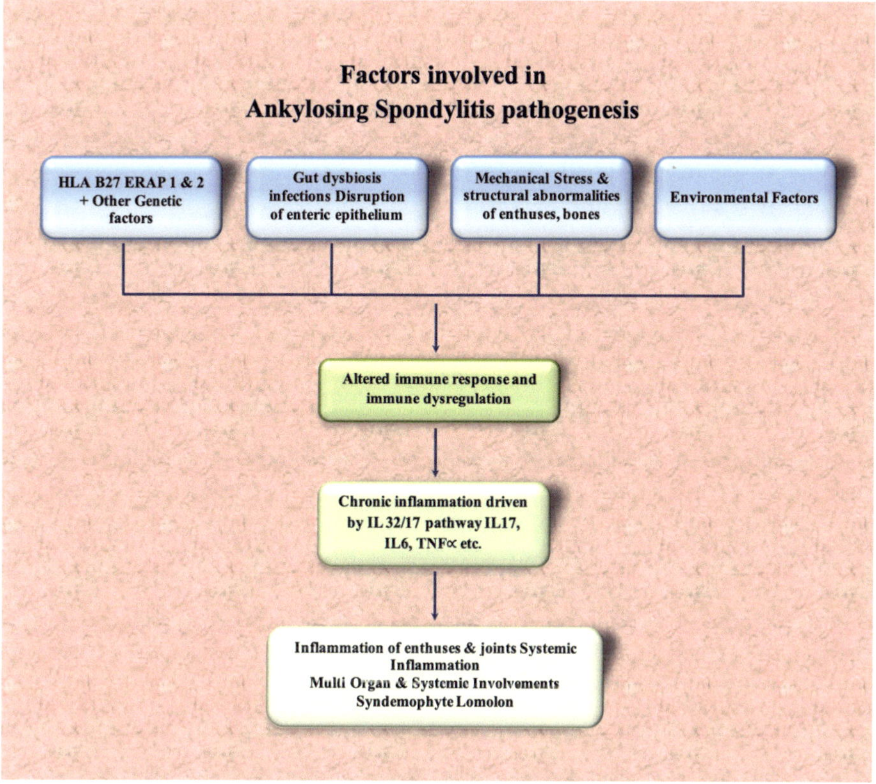

Figure 1.
Factors involved in ankylosing spondylitis pathogenesis.

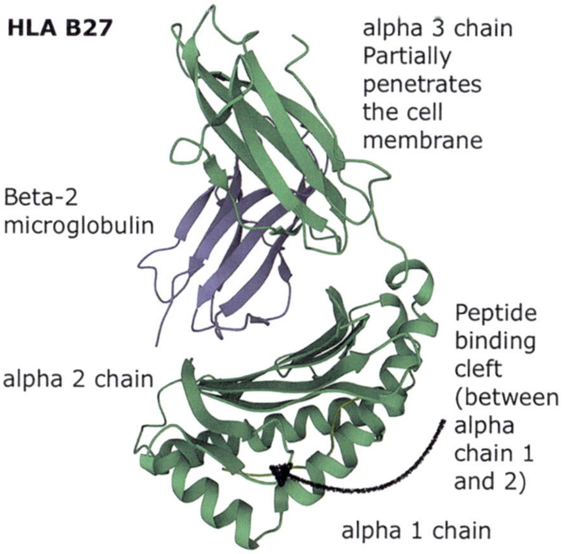

Figure 2.
HLA B27 protein structure [4, 5].

Extensive polymorphism of HLAB 27 results from the considerable variability of the heavy chain component of the protein [7].

Studies show 90–95% of AS patients are HLA-B27 positive. The chances of developing AS for an individual with an HLA-B27 gene is 1–2%. This percentage increases to 15–20% for those who have a first degree relative with AS [2]. The relative risk of developing AS for an individual with a first degree relative who has AS is 94%, for a second degree relative 25% and for a third degree relative 4% [2].

HLA B27 is a polymorphic gene with around 223 subtypes thus far identified [6]. HLAB2705 is more prevalent in affected Caucasians, HLAB2704 is associated with affected Han Chinese whilst HLAB2702 is associated with affected people of Mediterranean ethnicity [2]. HLA B2705 and HLA B2704 are the predominant subtypes in the South Indian population [8]. Inuit and native Alaskans have the highest rates of HLA B27 In the world and correspondingly the highest prevalence of AS [9].

Even though HLA B27 is the most commonly recognised genetic factor in the development of AS, its overall contribution in the development of AS is only around 20% suggesting other environmental, genetic, immune and even anatomical phenomena are responsible for pathogenesis in AS. For example, microRNAs (miRNAs) are a class of endogenous, non-coding, RNA-modulating mRNAs and are reported to regulate AS progression by interacting with genes that are potential biomarkers for AS [10].

2.1.2 Other HLA genes

Other HLA B genes have been recognised in association with development of AS including: HLA-B730 HLA-B16, HLA-B35,31,32 HLA-B38 and HLA-B3933 [2]. These genes have been identified across a variety of ethnic groups and are associated with HLA-B27-negative AS, although the mechanism is not yet clear [2].

An HLA-C amino-acid variant in addition to HLA-B*27 confers risk for ankylosing spondylitis in the Korean population. The four amino-acid positions of HLA-B and -C account for most of the associations between AS and MHC in the Korean population. This finding updates the list of AS susceptibility loci and provides new insight into AS pathogenesis mediated by MHC class I molecules [11].

2.1.3 ERAP1 ERAP2 and NPEPPS

ERAP1 (coding for endoplasmic reticulum aminopeptidase 1 (ERAP1)), ERAP2 (coding for ERAP2) and NPEPPS (coding for puromycin-sensitive aminopeptidase) have been implicated in AS [2]. This is to do with folding of HLA B27 in the endoplasmic reticulum which is discussed in further detail later on in this chapter. Gene–gene interactions between HLAB27 and ERAP1 appear to be responsible [2].

2.1.4 IL23R

More than 90% of genetic risk single nuclear polymorphisms (SNP)s are present in non-coding regions, however this is not the case with the IL23R gene. The genetic association of IL23R loci with AS was first reported in 2007. Interestingly, the same SNP also affects the risk of developing inflammatory bowel disease. The same SNP is also associated with psoriasis, another condition closely linked to AS [12].

2.1.5 Killer immunoglobulin-like receptor (KIRLR)

Studies have demonstrated that KIR3DL2 R is up-regulated on activated CD4+ T-cells and that there are increased levels of these cells in patients with AS compared with healthy controls [13]. These cells have been found upregulated in the terminal ilium of patients with early spondyloarthropathy [14]. The theories on the role of KIRLRs in AS are many with one suggesting an imbalance between inhibitory and excitatory KIR receptors in AS patients that upregulates an NK cell response [15].

2.1.6 Other genes

Over the years several genes have been reported in the literature in association with AS with new ones emerging as further research is undertaken.

Susceptibility genes have been identified that are either directly, or indirectly involved in the IL-23–IL-17 pathway, or interact with it in AS. These include IL12B, RUNX3, EOMES, TBX21, TYK2, CARD9, IL1R1, IL1R2, IL6R, IL7R, IL12B, IL27, NKX2 and PTGER4 [16]. The interleukin (IL)-1 gene cluster is an important locus associated with susceptibility to AS. CYP 2D6 [17] and ANKH genes are also associated with AS [18].

There is discussion around the association of TLR4 genetic variants and TLR4 expression levels with AS implicates innate immunity in AS pathogenesis 27,28. The concentrations of bacterial lipopolysaccharides (LPS) are increased in AS with further suggests the association with TLR4 expression and have been noted to correlate with disease activity [16]. This supports the concept that AS has autoinflammatory components in its pathophysiology.

Many more AS-susceptibility genes are likely to be identified by ongoing research.

2.1.7 Gene–gene interactions and pleiotropy

There are significant gaps in knowledge about gene–gene interactions and the development of AS. However, certain links have been established. For example, a Taiwanese population study is suggestive of an interaction between HLA-B60 and HLA-B27 as a marker for the risk of AS susceptibility [2]. The combination of HLA B60 with HLAB 27 increases chances of developing AS by 3–6 times. HLAB27 interacting with ERAP1 gene is thought to contribute to development of AS [19].

Pleiotropy in AS has been investigated. A number of pleotrophic gene loci have been identified [13]. DNA methylation genes 3a and 3b (*DNMT3A, DNM3TB*) are recognised in genomic imprinting and X-chromosome and have been studied in cross-gene studies. Their relationship with haematopoietic stem cell development and UBE2 activation (a family of genes also known to be associated with AS) supports the hypothesis of involvement in male predominance in AS, which remains currently remains unexplained [13].

FUT2 encodes fucosyl transferase, a gene which controls secretion of blood group antigens into body fluids. This gene is known has a major effect on the gut microbiome and is thought to contribute to AS [20].

It is likely that further research will illuminate several ways in which gene–gene interactions contribute in AS pathogenesis.

2.1.8 List of genes associated with ankylosing spondylitis

A list of genes associated with Ankylosing Spondylitis can be found by searching in the National Library of Medicine gene search engine at the following link: https://www.ncbi.nlm.nih.gov/gene/?term=Ankylosing+spondylitis

2.2 Immunological factors

The complex dynamic relationship involved with inflammatory cytokines in the development of AS includes the IL17/23 axis, which is the most well studied of these pathways, but IL6, IL10, IL22 and tumour necrosis factor are also recognised as contributing to chronic inflammation. Other inflammatory cytokines have been postulated as playing a role including IL37 [21], but the facts remain that the detailed mechanisms are unknown.

The differences observed in immune cells and cytokines in AS suggest an aberrant composition of immunological factors in AS pathogenesis. In the peripheral blood of AS patients and healthy HLA-B27-positive controls, for example, the levels of T cells secreting tumour necrosis factor (TNF)- α and interferon (IFN)-γ were reportedly lower. CD8+ T cells in AS patients tended to secrete more IL10 [2].

An abnormal polarisation of macrophages induced by IL-4 was found in AS patients [20]. Reports exist showing CD163+ macrophages are the predominant cells in inflamed peripheral joints in SpA patients [22].

Dendtritic cells (DCs) play a key role in ankylosing spondylitis. AS can develop in patients who receive bone marrow from donors with AS and it appears DCs are the drivers of AS development in these cases [22, 23]. Signalling pathways of DCs are dysregulated in ankylosing spondylitis with an associated Th17 inflammatory response [22]. One study identified patients with AS demonstrate altered DC and T cell populations implying pathogenic roles for the IL-23 cytokine axis in intestinal inflammation [24].

Patients with AS have significantly higher percentages of NK cells of the subset of CD56dim CD16+ [22]. This important immunologic characteristic in AS patients might explain the relationship between the autoinflammatory and autoimmune components of AS pathophysiology.

The term seronegative implies that the disease process does not have antibodies detected in serum antibody tests that are found in autoimmune conditions such as rheumatoid arthritis, SLE, primary Sjogren's Syndrome and scleroderma spectrum disorders, however emerging research has demonstrated an association of antibodies in AS [25–28]. As discussed, whilst AS might be initiated by the innate immune system with the connecting IL-17/23 pathway being prominent in the pathophysiology, there is known B cell activation and involvement of the adaptive immune system, so the generation of antibodies makes logical sense [25, 26]. Consensus on a distinct autoantibody is lacking, however this could emerge from ongoing research in the role of B cells in AS. The molecular mimicry hypothesis as demonstrated in patients with AS who have prior klebsiella and associated circulating antibodies also supports B cell involvement in AS [29].

Synovial biopsies of AS patients have been found to contain B-cell rich follicles with some literature reporting aggregates of T-cells and B-cells arranged into structures similar in appearance to germinal centres. However, the presence of lymphocytes has been argued as potentially being secondary recruitment to an already established inflammatory processes [30]. This introduces debate in literature on whether AS is autoinflammatory in nature rather than autoimmune, with the truth being more complex than a mere dichotomous linear continuum of possibilities.

Innate lymphoid cells are also recognised to play an important role in AS. ILC3 cells in particular are thought to be involved in the pathogenesis of inflammation. They reside in the gut and express the alpha-4/beta-7 integrin, functions as a homing receptor. In patients with AS the ligand for this particular integrin, mucosal vascular addressin cell adhesion molecule 1 (MADCAM1), is more strongly expressed in high endothelial venules (HEV) of the intestines, the blood, synovium and also in bone marrow [31]. One theory postulates that these IL-17+ and IL-22+ ILC3 cells migrate from the gut into the systemic circulation and via integrin-ligand communication are drawn towards target tissues in the bone marrow, joints, peripheral joints, and entheses [31].

The roll of T cells in ankylosing spondylitis drives the immunological response in AS. A large range of T cells are involved. Th17 cells secrete IL-17 which is one of the main inflammatory cytokines involved in AS. A list of T cells involved with AS is provided in **Table 1**.

Strong evidence suggests a central role of IL-17 secreting γδ T cells in the pathogenesis of AS [32]. These cells have been found to be present in increased numbers in the blood of AS patients, but have also been identified as resident cells within entheses [32]. It is thought that microtrauma and mechanical loading of the entheses activates resident immune cells that trigger an aberrant immune response in AS.

T reg cells are known to be dysfunctional in AS. FOXP3+ T reg cells have been described in AS [15, 33]. FOXP3+ is a protein that is affected by hormonal fluctuations, inflammatory cytokines and danger signals and it is thought that this possibly accounts for some of the gender bias in AS presentation as well as other autoimmune disorders [33].

IL-17 positive mucosal-associated invariant T (MAIT) cells are one of the subsets of innate-like cells and are elevated in AS patients, particularly in synovial fluid, but also in circulating blood [34].

Cells that are major components in the immunological response in AS patients are summarised in **Table 1** [1, 22].

2.3 Infections and microbiome

The human enteric system contains unique microbiota with a stable ecology and dynamic equilibrium [35]. This association between host and symbiotic microbes is the result of millions of years of coevolution leading to homeostatic equilibrium between enteric flora and host health and disease [35–37]. The composition of an individuals' microbiota is generally highly resistant to change, however is influenced by a range of exogenous factors. The resilience of this complex adaptive system is impacted by major perturbations, which can lead to a 'tipping point' beyond with significant change can occur and disease might result [36]. Studies in metabolomics demonstrate small-molecule metabolites generated from microbiota can influence intestinal inflammation, and potentially result in joint inflammation [38] and the development of AS [20]. Furthermore, the enteric microbiome of patients with AS has been shown to exhibit a higher load of bacterial peptides known to be presented by HLA-B27 [20]. This suggests either HLA-B27 fails to clear these, or that these peptides drive the immune response associated with HLA-B27, a potentially important

Cell Type	Function	Alteration in AS
CD14–CD16+ Dendritic cells	Interacts with HLAB27, induces the IL23/27 pathway Secretes IL-6 and IL-1β	Increased
CD 163+ Macrophages	Secretes IL23	Increased
CD56dim CD16+ NK cells	Interacts with HLAB27 via KIR3DL1/3DS1 locus	Increased
Th1 helper cells (CD4+ subset)	Secretes (IFN-γ), IL- 2, and tumour necrosis factor alpha (TNF-α)	Increased
Th2 helper cells	Secretes IL4, IL10, IL13	Increased
Thl7 cells (CD4+ subset) (5 different types IL-17A, IL-17B, IL-17C, IL-17D, IL-17E, IL-17F)	Secretes IL17 in AS also secretes IL6, IL IL-26, IFN-γ	Increased
Thl/Th2 and Thl7/Treg	Promotes IL17 pathway	Increased ratio
T22 cells (CD4+ subset)	Secretes IL-22, IL-13, and TNF-α	Increased
TCD3+ TCD8+ cells	Differentiate into Tc1 and Tcl7 generating TNF-α, IFN-γ and IL-17 and driving inflammatory pathway as well as lysing cells via perforin/ granzyme or signalling through Fas/ FasL pathway	Increased
CD19+, CD86+,CD95+,CD27-B cells	Ectopic lymphoid structures in joints	Increased
IL-17+ Mucosal-associated invariant T (MAIT) cells	Secrete IL17, IL 22 and IFN-γ	Increased
Innate lymphoid cells	ILC1 secretes IFN-γ	Increased levels of ILC3 cells in peripheral blood
	ILC2 is the main source of IL-4, IL-5, and IL-9;	
	ILC3 secretes IL-17 and IL-22 in response to IL-23	
γδT cells (T cell subset) 50% of cell types at mucosal and epithelial sites	Produce IL17	Increased levels in peripheral blood as well as in entheses

Table 1.
Some alterations to pro-inflammatory cells in AS.

finding in the role of understanding the relationship between gut dysregulation, HLA B27 and AS [20].

The 'joint-gut' axis is a term used to describe the relationship between microbiome dysregulation inflammation and musculoskeletal manifestations in AS and other autoimmune diseases [39]. The 'leaky gut' allows bacteria derived proteins and primed immune cells into systemic circulation eliciting a systemic immune response. However, several challenges exist in establishing the role specific microorganisms play in gut dysbiosis. Firstly, the concept of an organism being pathogenic as opposed to commensal flora is largely context dependent. Secondly, establishing causation as opposed to association remains problematic [36]. Thirdly, there is the challenge of establishing whether there exists a characteristic microbiome that is specific to AS patients (**Figure 3**) [40].

Many of these microbes were thought to be gut commensals, but new studies have shown them to be increased specifically with disease and thus are regarded as pathobiont [36].

Despite this there exists a large volume of literature demonstrating distinct changes in the microbiome of patients with AS. Experimental models of AS have attempted to describe causal microbial pathways, but this is an ongoing endeavour in research. For example, decreased numbers of Firmicutes, particularly the species *Faecalibacterium prausnitzii* and also *Clostridium leptum* have been found in spondyloathrtidites and inflammatory bowel disease (IBD) and present an important link between the seronegative spondyloarthropathies (SpA) and gut inflammation [36]. *Porphyromonas gingivalis*, a periodontal bacterium, with an ability to colonise synovial joints and exacerbate collagen-induced arthritis in mouse models [41].

Various reports estimate up to 70 percent of patients with HLA-B27-associated spondylarthritis have microscopic gut lesions [20], with around one third demonstrating overt gut inflammation [42]. First degree relatives of these patients show signs of subclinical gut inflammation and impaired gut epithelial barrier [43]. Importantly, the degree of enteric inflammation correlates with disease activity and degree of sacroiliac (SI) joint inflammation [42].

Dialister is a saccharolytic bacteria, belongs to family *Vellionelaceae*. One study demonstrated inflamed intestinal tissue contained higher levels of this bacteria compared to non-inflamed tissue and correlated with increased disease scores in AS patients [44].

Ruminococcus gnavus is a known pathobiont associated both spondyloarthritis and inflammatory bowel disease [38].

A Chinese study on AS patients showed elevated numbers of *Akkermansia muciniphila* and several *Prevotella* species, including Prevotella *melaninogenica, Prevotella copri*, and *Prevotella* spp. all of which are mucin degrading bacteria along with *Bifidobacterium* whilst reduced *Bacteroides* species were noted [45].

Increased abundance of *Mucispirillum schaedleri* is thought to possibly compromise the spatial segregation by bringing luminal microbes closer to the intestinal epithelial cells which induces and inflammatory response [36].

IgA coated *E coli* have been shown to induce IL17 inflammation and correspond with increased disease activity scores in patients with spondyloarthritis and Crohn's Disease [46].

The role of fungal agents in enteric dysbiosis is being investigated. Fungal bioproducts including β-glucan are thought to trigger AS in certain mouse models [36]. IL-17 inhibitors has demonstrated a shift in bacterial and fungal composition of the enteric microbiome in patients. Anti-*Saccharomyces cerevisiae* antibodies are associated with intestinal inflammation in patients with Axial spondyloarthritis and Chron's disease according to one study [47]. In such studies biome disturbances result in overexpression of IL-17/23 cytokines and the expansion of IL-25/17 [48].

Recent studies have examined the role of inter-kingdom fungal-bacterial interactions in AS patients revealing perturbed relations including decreased fungal to bacterial biodiversity ratios in these patients [49].

The human gut virome has also gained attention, however has remained a particularly challenging area with limited studies. It is thought to modulate the bacteriome via bacteriophages [36, 50]. *Caudovirales* bacteriophages are reported to be increased in Crohn's Disease. In the healthy gut the viral core reportedly consists of virulent

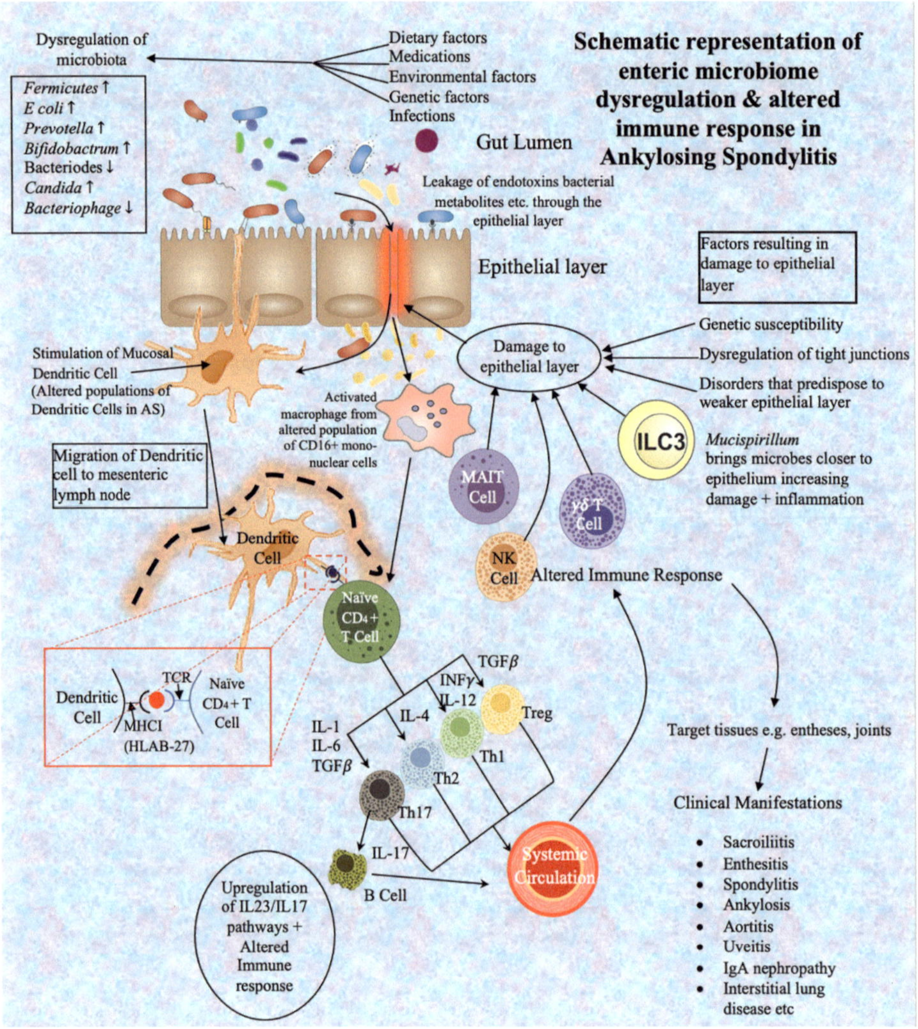

Figure 3.
Schematic representation of enteric microbiome dysregulation & altered immune response in ankylosing spondylitis.

phages. However, in patients with Crohn's Disease, the virome shifts towards a less virulent bacteriophage core that correspondingly affects the bacterial community and encourages infection [36].

The role of infection in development of spondyloarthritis and AS specifically is well documented in medical literature. Research demonstrates infections significantly increase the risks of AS [51].

Cases of reactive arthritis (ReA) following venereal infection date back to the early 1800s [52]. Approximately 12–16% of individuals who initially present with ReA go onto develop AS. Patients who are HLAB27 positive have a worse prognosis, however it is still unclear whether infection is the provoking factor in patients who develop AS in this context, or whether these patients would have developed AS anyway [53]. The pathophysiological mechanisms between ReA and development of AS have not been identified, however it is postulated that chronic infections result in altered immunological response resulting in arthritis. Research demonstrates the presence of yersinia in the lymph nodes of those with *Yersinia* related arthritis and *Chlamydia* in the synovial fluids and tissue of those with chronic seronegative arthritis [54].

Gram negative infections in the gut are particularly associated with spondyloarthritis and reactive arthritis with chronic infections conferring a greater risk of progression to AS. (*Shigella, Salmonella, Yersinia,* are known to produce inflammatory arthritis as are *Campylobacter* species, *Clostridium difficile, Brucella,* and *Giardia* [6, 20].

The antigen-binding region of several HLAB27 genotypic subtypes, especially HLA B2705 share an amino acid sequence with nitrogenase from Klebsiella *pneumoniae*. This has led to a theory that molecular mimicry following certain infections is a possible mechanism for pathogenesis of AS in genetically susceptible hosts [29].

HLA-B27 results in a robust cytotoxic CD8+ T cell response to certain viruses, including hepatitis C, influenza and HIV, therefore it is possible that HLAB27 actually confers an evolutionary advantage in certain infectious contexts [55]. Research has demonstrated that HLA molecules can affect the severity and duration of viral infection [56]. Case reports of Sars-2-cov infection capable of triggering a reactive arthritis and uveitis in an HLA B27 positive patient exists [57, 58]. Other research suggests that Sars 2-Cov might have a predilection for people with certain HLA phenotypes [59]. The relationship between these various phenomena and the subsequent development of AS is an area which is likely to emerge in ongoing research and has important implications for both rheumatology and infectious diseases.

Prior flu infection may influence the presentation of such arthritogenic peptides especially in the presence of individuals with both ERAP1 and HLAB27 genes [3].

2.4 Metabolomics

Studies on metabolomics have gained attention in recent years. This has relevance to understanding pathogenesis, diagnosis and response to treatment in AS [60].

Studies show a range of findings in AS patients including altered pathways of tryptophan metabolism [61]. Other studies revealed significant alterations in unsaturated fatty acids (FA), linoleic acid, alpha-linolenic acid, FA degradation, and FA biosynthesis pathways [9].

One study on AS metabolomics noted alterations in several pathways including amino acid biosynthesis, glycolysis, glutaminolysis, fatty acids biosynthesis and choline metabolism developed a diagnostic panel comprising five metabolites (L-glutamate, arachidonic acid, L-phenylalanine, PC (18:1(9Z)/18:1(9Z)), 1-palmitoylglycerol). This study found that TNF inhibitors treatment could restore the equilibrium of 21 metabolites [62]. Another study revealed down regulation of the Vitamin D3 metabolite—(23S,25R)-25-hydroxyvitamin D3 26,23-peroxylactone. The ratio this vitamin D metabolite *versus* vitamin D binding protein serum levels was shown to be altered when compared with healthy controls [63].

2.5 Sex hormones

Until recently it was thought that a relationship between male gender and presence of AS existed, given males account for the majority of AS patients, however recent literature demonstrates a more homogenous sex prevalence of AS [64]. Although this is true, females with AS have different phenotypical disease due to different immunological, hormonal, and genetic responses [64].

One study examining the differences between manifestations of AS in male vs. female patients demonstrated different levels of TNF, proinflammatory cytokines IL-6, IL-17, and IL-18. These authors noted a longer diagnostic delay in female AS patients compared to males. Several studies have reported female AS patients experience a higher number of extra-articular manifestations (EAM) including inflammatory bowel disease, enthesitis, psoriasis, whereas EAMs are less common in male patients with the exception of anterior uveitis which occurs more frequently in males with AS [64]. Radiographic damage and progression of disease is worse in male patients [64].

Despite this these recognised relationships, the role of sex hormones and biologic gender in AS pathogenesis remains poorly understood [65]. This is complicated by conflicting evidence in research to date [66] with a lack of robust study design to date [67].

A small study by Odeh *et al.* [66] reported spinal syndesmophyte scores do not correlate with testosterone levels. One study suggested testosterone, in particular, attenuates inflammatory processes via a number of cellular and molecular pathways [68].

However, some reports on variations of sex hormones in AS patients compared with controls imply that increased androgen levels in both males and females possibly contributes to disease development [69]. Patients who are HLA-B27 were originally reported to have higher levels of testosterone [70]. However, a study with small sample size revealed a decreased testicular testosterone reserve, elevated luteinizing hormone level, and inversion of the normal estradiol/testosterone ratio and increased estradiol level [2]. In female studies reports show that patients with active AS have significantly lower estradiol levels in the menstrual period. Case reports of increase in incidence post pregnancy also suggest that sex hormones play a role with a proposed hypothalamic–pituitary–adrenal axis impairment [2].

One study demonstrated that SKG MICE who received oestrogen therapy showed little inflammatory infiltrates of Achilles tendon, or spinal discs compared with mice who had undergone oophorectomy [71]. One report proposed ostrogens might reduce arthritis due to their suppression of wnt signalling [72]. Another study reported that selective oestrogen receptor modulator (SERM) lasofoxifene not only suppresses the effects of joint inflammation and improves bone mineral density in SKG mice, but it also affected the composition and biodiversity of the gut microbiome, with the authors concluding further reaserch on the role of SERMS to evaluate their effects in SpA is required [73].

There is literature to suggest a relationship between women who experience excess androgen levels in conditions such as polycystic ovarian syndrome (PCOS) and development of AS [74], as well as other rheumatic diseases [75]. A Korean study questioned whether other factors besides sex hormones play a role in reduced disease progression in females noting in their study there was no significant relationship between oestrogen levels and radiographic progression [73].

This research into excess androgen levels in some AS patients has led to researchers in the past asking the question whether patients who are HLA-B27 positive would benefit from anti-androgen therapy [76]. However this remains to be addressed by research with some emerging literature demonstrating progression of ankylosis in mouse models where anti-androgen therapy has been used to treat excess androgen levels [65].

There is growing recognition of the relationship between metabolic syndrome and ankylosing spondylitis [77–79], with one Morrocon study demonstrating a prevalence of 34% and a male predominance of 67% [80] Another study demonstrated treatment with anti-TNF-α monoclonal antibody infliximab reversed excess insulin levels in non-diabetic patients [77]. It is possible to postulate that there might be a relationship between androgen excess metabolic syndrome and the development of AS, but this relationship requires more research to establish.

Of note is the incidence among men and women is similar in non-radiographic axial spondyloarthropathy, ie in individuals meeting clinical criteria for axial spondyloarthritis without radiological evidence of sacroiliitis on x rays [2].

It should be noted that most studies conducted in this area are of small sample size only, or have been performed in animal models. It is known that immune responses due to sex differences change throughout the life of an individual and are influenced by age and reproductive status and that sex hormones impact on different immune responses between the sexes [81]. Additionally, it is now recognised that environmental factors including microbiome composition and nutrional status impact immunological response differently in males and females [81]. Therefore it appears likely that additional endocrinological, immunological, genetic and environmental factors interacting with sex hormones contribute to pathogenesis of AS. Further research is required to better understand this complex relationship.

2.6 Diet and lifestyle factors

Currently evidence on the relationship between AS and diet is extremely limited and inconclusive. This is mainly due to studies being small, single studies with moderate-to-high risk of bias, and insufficient reporting of results as reported by one systematic review [82].

No prospective cohort studies of dietary risk factors for the development of AS exist, however one report suggested that a change in dietary habit from a high protein, low-starch diet to a Westernised high-starch diet among the Inuit population of Alaska and Canada whose populations also express high percentages of HLA B-27, possibly explain an increased incidence of AS in this population [83]. Other studies have suggested adoption of a "Westernised" diet is a contributing factor to development of AS [84]. One study reported that patients with AS were breastfed less compared with healthy controls [85]. Breast feeding could potentially affect the development of AS through microbiome and other immunological factors.

Mouse models demonstrated that those with a high salt diet resulted in significantly higher Th17 in their gut lamina propria [86]. Human studies revealed males who were fed a high salt diet increased the Th17 cells in their peripheral blood and demonstrated a corresponding loss of lactobacillus species [86].

Smoking is associated with increased cumulative spinal structural damage in patients with AS [87] as well as higher disease activity, inflammatory markers and functional disability [88]. Whether smoking induces AS is unclear.

Alcohol consumption is associated with spinal structural progression in patients with axial spondyloarthritis and appears to be dose related according to one Korean study [89]. These researchers demonstrated an increase of syndesmophyte progression over a two-year period.

2.7 Environmental factors

A report demonstrated significantly higher urine concentrations of cadmium, antimony, tungsten, uranium, and trimethylarsine in patients with AS compared to healthy controls [90].

Whilst there is very limited research on the role of other environmental toxins and development of AS in the literature, there is a well-established ongoing discussion on the role of a range of environmental toxins in the development of autoimmune diseases [91, 92]. Alterations to the gut biome through interference by toxic substances is one proposed mechanism [93]. Further research is required to establish whether any chemical contributions play a role in the pathogenesis of AS. This includes examining whether endocrine disrupting chemicals, pesticides and other substances might impact the immune-endocrine axis of patients with any genetic susceptibility to developing AS.

2.8 Anatomic factors

Structural integrity of anatomical in patients could possibly predispose certain individuals to the development of AS. For example, it is known that mucosal integrity plays in important role in gut dysbiosis and factors that weaken the mucosal layer predispose to enteric inflammation and possible generation of aberrant immune pathways. It is possible to assume, therefore that disorders resulting in fragile mucosa would also potentially generate an increased risk of permeability, inflammation and associated arthritis. One report revealed circulating levels of connective tissue degradation are diagnostic and prognostic markers in AS [94]. At a microscopic level, barrier integrity of the intestinal mucosa is maintained by intestinal epithelial tight junction proteins. These include occludin, claudins, and zonula occludens. Where dysfunction of these proteins occur this could affect the tight junctions. This is proposed as a contributory mechanism by which microorganisms and their products penetrate the gut wall with associated activation of mucosal inflammation [95].

Clinical studies in patients with AS suggest there is involvement with mechanical strain and inflammation of the entheses [1] with a tendency for normal inflammatory and repair pathways to go awry in the context of AS.

Patients with conditions that potentially affect the strength and quality of these tissues might be at an increased risk of developing AS through altered responses to normal loads and associated immunological response. This means it is possible that patients who have conditions of heritable disorders of connective tissue (HDCT) to have weaker tissues that predispose them to development AS and might account for comorbid case reports in the literature, but other contributory factors including HLA-B27 might also be responsible. For example, one study reported 24% of patients with hypermobile Ehlers Danlos Syndrome (H-EDS) were positive for HLA-B27 [96]. Case reports of EDS and comorbid ankylosing spondylitis exist [97–101]. Further research is warranted to quantify this interesting connection that might provide key information on the pathophysiology in certain subsets of patients of patients with AS.

Eighty percent of tendons are comprised of collagen with type collagen 1 accounting for 60–85% of the total [51]. Disorders affecting collagen could contribute to the pathogenesis of AS. However, there might be evidence against this theory. One study revealed higher levels of both COL1A1 and RUNX2 in the AS ligament tissues than in non-AS ligament tissues [10]. Further research is required to clarify this relationship.

2.9 Racial/ethnic differences

The relationship between various ethnicities and prevalence of the HLA-B27 gene as well as development of AS, is well reported in the literature. Between 10 to 16% of Norwegians, Swedes and Icelanders are positive for HLA-B27 and between 25 to 50%

of Inuit, Yupik and Indigenous Northern Americans [102]. Ankylosing spondylitis is three times less common in American blacks than in whites. It is extremely rare in African blacks of unmixed ancestry [103]. A histocompatibility antigen HLA-B27, which does not exist in African blacks of unmixed ancestry, and is present in eight percent of white and two to four percent of the American black population, is strongly associated with ankylosing spondylitis and Reiter's disease [103]. HLA-B27 is present in more than 80 percent of white patients with ankylosing spondylitis or Reiter's disease but in less than 60 percent of American black patients [103]. HLA-B27 occurred in 62.5% of African Americans, 85.3% of White Americans, and 86.7% of Americans with Latino ethnicity ($p < 0.0001$). Higher disease activity scores have been associated with an American black ethnicity. African Americans with AS have more severe disease compared to either White Americans, or Latinos [104]. This could be partially influenced by social determinants of health.

3. Pathophysiology

Key aspects in ankylosing (AS) pathophysiology are well understood, however the overarching network of immunological dysregulation is exceptionally complex and remains elusive despite extensive research.

Broadly speaking the pathophysiological processes within AS can be considered as musculoskeletal (articular, osteo and entheses-related) and extra articular (ocular, enteric, renal, pulmonary, vascular and dermatological).

Within the musculoskeletal aspects of AS, three major features of the disease exist. Inflammation of the joint and entheses, significant bone demineralisation and ossification of characteristic joints and entheses.

The extra-articular pathophysiological processes involved in AS are poorly understood and are not the major focus of this chapter.

The chronic inflammation in AS results in fibrosis and ossification and ultimately a fused spine with the characteristic bamboo spine seen on xray imaging Inflammatory responses involved include CD4+ and CD8+ T lymphocytes and macrophages, cytokines, particularly tumour necrosis factor-α (TNF-α) and transforming growth factor-β (TGF-β). The IL-23/IL-17 axis is recognised as the principle driving immunological force responsible for perpetuation of the chronic inflammation with Th17 cells and the production of the proinflammatory cytokine IL-17 playing a central role in the process [105].

There has been debate in the literature on whether AS is an autoinflammatory condition, or an autoimmune disease [16]. Autoinflammatory diseases are primarily driven by the innate immune system and, whilst autoimmune diseases are driven by the adaptive immune system and primarily present as a B cell response. Literature examining the role of the innate immune system communicating with the adaptive immune system has led some researchers to recommend that autoinflammation and autoimmunity should not be considered as opposing mechanisms, but rather as extreme opposites of a continuum, with different combinations and permutations resulting in specific clinical phenotypes [15, 16]. Whilst conceptually it is possible to separate aspects of immunological responses for the purposes of discussion and research, *in vivo* particularly with regards to AS, the situation is a complex symphony of enmeshed networks between adaptive and innate pathways that remain to be fully understood. These processes should be considered interlinked non-linear matrices rather than 2 systems on a dichotomous spectrum.

Genetic studies support the role of auto inflammation in AS pathophysiology. Research on Turkish and Iranian individuals reported a significant association between variants of MEFV and the risk of developing AS. MEFV is a gene that encodes for pyrin which is a recognised promoter of autoinflammation. Comorbidities of spondyloarthritides are reported in association with familial Mediterranean Fever [16], whilst there is discussion in the literature on the relationship between Behcet's Disease and AS although there are also reports of a relation. A theory has emerged on the concept of an overarching 'MCH-1-opathy' that accounts for the possible shared pathophysiology between the seronegative spondyloarthropathies and Behcet's Disease [23].

In the 1980s there was literature published discussing an apparent increase in responsiveness to complement activators in diseases associated with HLA-B27 [106]. There is now an emerging body of literature examining the role of compliment in AS [107–109]. The complement system is a cascade of protein cleaving resulting in a powerful pro inflammatory response. Complement is capable of destroying invading pathogens, however when there is dysregulation of complement including uncontrolled activation of the cascade combined with insufficient regulation, the destructive capabilities against invading pathogens turn against host cells. There are several studies in the literature demonstrating elevated complement products C3, C4 and C3d IgA, IgG, C-reactive protein (CRP), serum amyloid A, apolipoprotein A in AS patients [110, 111]. Circulating immune complexes have been reportedly higher in AS [112]. Additionally, reports that tumour necrosis factor inhibitors appear to reduce complement levels and reduction in arthrogenesis [108] suggest the complement cascade might be a contributing factor in the pathophysiology of AS. It is possible through this mechanism extra articular manifestations of AS including amyloidosis and IgA vasculitis might be triggered although there are reports that the manitose binding lectin levels are decreased in patients with AS which goes against this theory [113]. Infection with Klebsiella is recognised as being a significant complement cascade activator via cross-reactive antibodies against autoantigens in the infective process [107].

3.1 The IL17/23 pathway and HLA B27

There are several theories on the involvement of HLA-B27s involvement in the IL17/23 pathway. Despite this, the exact mechanisms and relationship between inflammation and resulting clinical signs of ankylosis are not fully elucidated and there is acknowledgment of knowledge gaps that remain problematic in much published research.

HLA-B27's functional role is in peptide presentation to cytotoxic T cells and NK cells. Within the endoplasmic reticulum (ER) of the antigen presenting cell, HLA-B27 binds short peptides which are then trafficked to the cell surface via the golgi apparatus and displayed ready for presentation to other immunological cells [54]. In the case of AS it is thought that HLA-B27s role in triggering the immune system might occur through different pathways. Several theories exist around how HLA-B27 results in an aberrant immunological response in the context of AS.

Firstly, protein misfolding in the ER accumulate generating ER stress that generates upregulation of IL-17 and other proinflammatory cytokines. HLA-B27 must fold and bind with protein β2m in the ER. This process is slow in HLA-B27 especially in the case of misfolding resulting in increased oxidation and formation of disulphide linked homodimers [114]. ER stress results from an inability of the ER to remove misfolded proteins resulting in what is known as the "unfolded protein response" (UPR) essentially a gain of function response. Degradation of abnormal proteins is regulated by ERAD pathway. This can result in a loss of function [7].

In extreme instances the accumulation of aberrant HLA-B27 results in apoptosis. It is theorised that the UPR results in upregulation of IL-12/via the transcription factor CHOP 23 [115]. In rat models UPR produces an up regulation of TNF alpha and ILS which results in an overall osteoclastogenesis response [115] and accounts for bone demineralisation seen in AS.

The ER stress response is also thought to be the reason behind the association of ERAP1 gene in AS pathogenesis both in HLA-B27 positive and negative patients. Whilst ERAP1 is primarily found in the ER it is also secreted by macrophages and activated by INF-gamma and lipopolysaccharides. ERAP1 is responsible for protein trimming in the ER and altered genes can contribute to the production of aberrant proteins in the HLA-B27 production pathway [115].

Although there is conflicting evidence in current research, some literature proposes quantitative changes in the peptide composition in AS and that an 'arthritogenic peptide repertoire' could contribute to AS pathogenesis [54]. NK cell receptors can recognise MHC class I molecules in addition to TCR recognition. This includes HLA-B27, and the reciprocal receptor for HLA-B27 heterotrimers KIR3DL1, has been shown to be sensitive to certain properties of peptides bound to HLA-B27 [116, 117]. Therefore, it is possible that alterations in these peptides could affect immune responses via KIR signalling [54].

Changes in this peptide repertoire could potentially affect misfolding and free heavy chain, or homodimer expression and contribute to this aspect of pathogenesis in AS [54]. A Trimolecular complex comprised of a B27 heavy chain, α2 microglobulin and a third peptide of either HLA-B27, a free heavy chain, or homodimers of HLA-B27, can possibly be recognized as neoantigens by the T cell receptor on CD4+ T cells leading to an autoimmune response [118–120].

The third theory around aberrant HLA-B27 is that misfolded HLA-B27 heavy chains are expressed on the cell surface as homodimers are responsible for an increased Th17 response via stimulation of the killer immunoglobulin receptor on natural killer (NK cells) and T cells which then drive an IL17 inflammatory response [54].

An additional theory with evidence is that dendritic cells exhibiting aberrant HLA-B27 result in loss of immune tolerance and development of autoimmunity [54].

Finally, it is postulated that certain microorganisms and cross-reactive epitopes might alter HLA27, but also that HLA-B27 itself exerts an effect on the composition of gut flora (**Figure 4**) [121].

IL-23 and IL-12 are cytokines that act as a bridge between the innate and adaptive branches of the immune system. Their critical and central role in AS is possible evidence that AS is both an autoinflammatory and autoimmune disease. The intestines are the major site of production of IL-23 [39]. HLA-B27 is thought to play a major role in IL23 and IL-12 production via the theories discussed in the previous section and the dendric cell is the primary cell that secretes these in the context of AS.

Studies on the role of IL-23 in ankylosing spondylitis demonstrates the IL-23/IL-17 axis is a non-linear matrix of complex pathways displaying overlapping yet distinct pathobiology [122]. Despite this, some research reveals that blocking the IL-17 pathway does not prevent the progression of ankylosing spondylitis [122].

IL-12 induces INF-γ which drives inflammation in AS. δγT cells and innate lymphoid cells exhibit the IL-23 receptor demonstrating their first line response to IL-23 [39]. However, Th0 cells and CD4+ cells do not exhibit an IL-23 receptor and require prior stimulation with a range of proinflammatory cytokines to become responsive to IL-23. These include IL1β and a range of other proinflammatory cytokines. Once activated via IL-23, αβT cells, δγT cells and innate lymphoid cells secrete

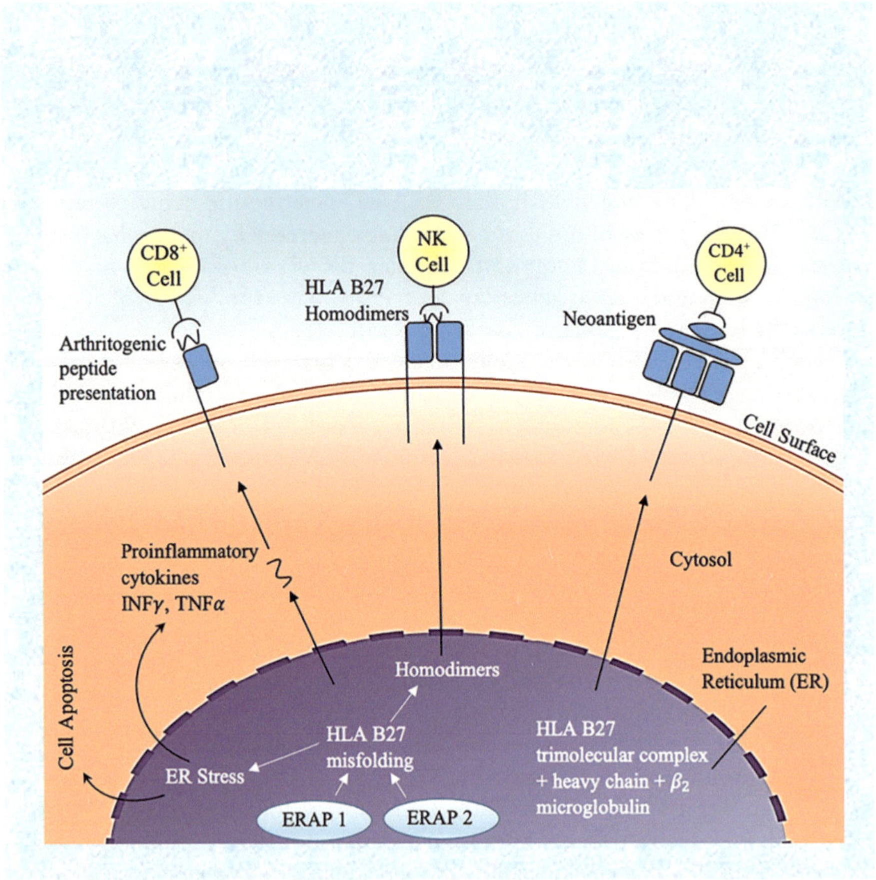

Figure 4.
Proposed theories on the role of HLA B27 & ERAP genes in pathogenesis of ankylosing spondylitis.

a range of proinflammatory cytokines including IL-17, IL-22, TNF-α and moreover αβT cells become unresponsive to the suppressive activity of T reg cells [39]. δ γT cells and innate lymphoid cells play a major role in the pathophysiology of AS [32]. Dysfunctional regulatory T cell behaviour has been identified in AS and has been associated with a loss of Tim-3, a member of the novel Tim (T cell immunoglobulin and mucin domain) family [123, 124].

T cells without IL-23 receptors exhibit IL-12Rβ1 receptors that are responsive to IL-12. Intracellular pathways involving Janus Kinase 2 (JAK2) and Tyrosine Kinase 2 (TYK2) produce STAT 4 and STAT 3 phosphorylation respectively resulting in a product ophan receptor gamma tau (RORγτ) which is essential for development of Th17 cells that ultimately drive the IL-17 aspect of this pathway (**Figure 5**) [125].

IL-17 is produced via a variety of mechanisms in AS. The IL-23 pathway discussed above leads to activation of T CD8+ cells, NK T cells and δγT cells all of which secrete IL-17, however in AS the major secreters of IL-17 come from CD4+ Th17 cells [39]. IL-17 plays a major role in the recruitment of neutrophils via IL-6 [1]. IL-17 also activates osteoclasts and directly stimulates B cells which are thought to form germinal centres in AS [26].

Pro-inflammatory cytokines critical drivers of the chronic inflammation in AS. IL-17F has recently been proposed to contribute to the pathobiology of both

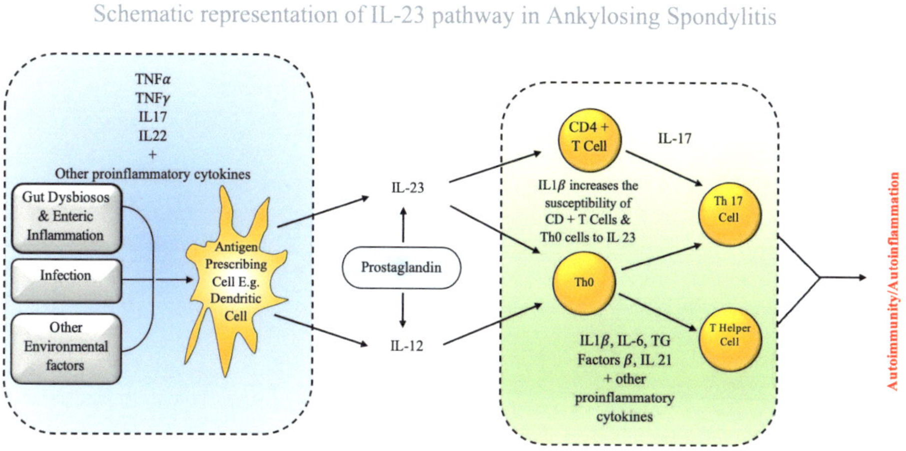

Figure 5.
Schematic representation of IL 23 pathway in ankylosing spondylitis.

inflammation and new bone formation in spondyloarthritis. Other inflammatory cytokines are also thought to contribute to chronic inflammation including granulocyte colony stimulating factor (G-CSF) raising the possibility of research into targeting upstream activators of Th17 cells rather than IL-17 itself (**Figure 6**) [122].

3.2 Bone Remodelling in AS

Molecular mechanisms underlying the extra-articular bone formation in patients with AS remain poorly understood. Mechanical factors including repetition and overload are regarded as contributing factors.

Dickkopf-related protein 1 (Dkk-1) and sclerostin levels, with a corresponding increase in the wnt pathway have been reported in AS [87]. TGFβ signalling pathway, Hedgehog signalling pathway, hypoxic cell signalling pathway are all reported to contribute to ossification [51]. Studies indicate the Wnt pathway appears to be a major factor in the dual relationship between new bone formation and bone loss in found in AS. Observed decreased serum levels of both Dkk-1 and sclerostin, suggest a link between excessive Wnt exposure and the new focal bone formation. There has been a negative association between Dkk-1, spinal BMD, and vertebral fractures reported in one study [126]. One report noted conflicting evidence in the literature on the role of Dkk-1 in AS offering the opinion this could partly be explained by variations in PTH and vitamin D and the fact vitamin D metabolism is impaired in inflammatory disease [72].

Evidence exists supporting theories on activation of bone morphogenetic protein signalling and a decrease in bone remodelling in AS [127].

The link between inflammation of the entheses and ossification, particularly within the annulus fibrosis with characteristic syndesmophyte formation in ankylosing spondylitis remains contentious. It is a non-linear and complex process. Some research suggests new bone formation may progress independently of the inflammatory process, and may even be accelerated by the resolution of inflammation [128].

Pathological bone remodelling in AS thought to be fundamentally different from physiological bone turnover [127].

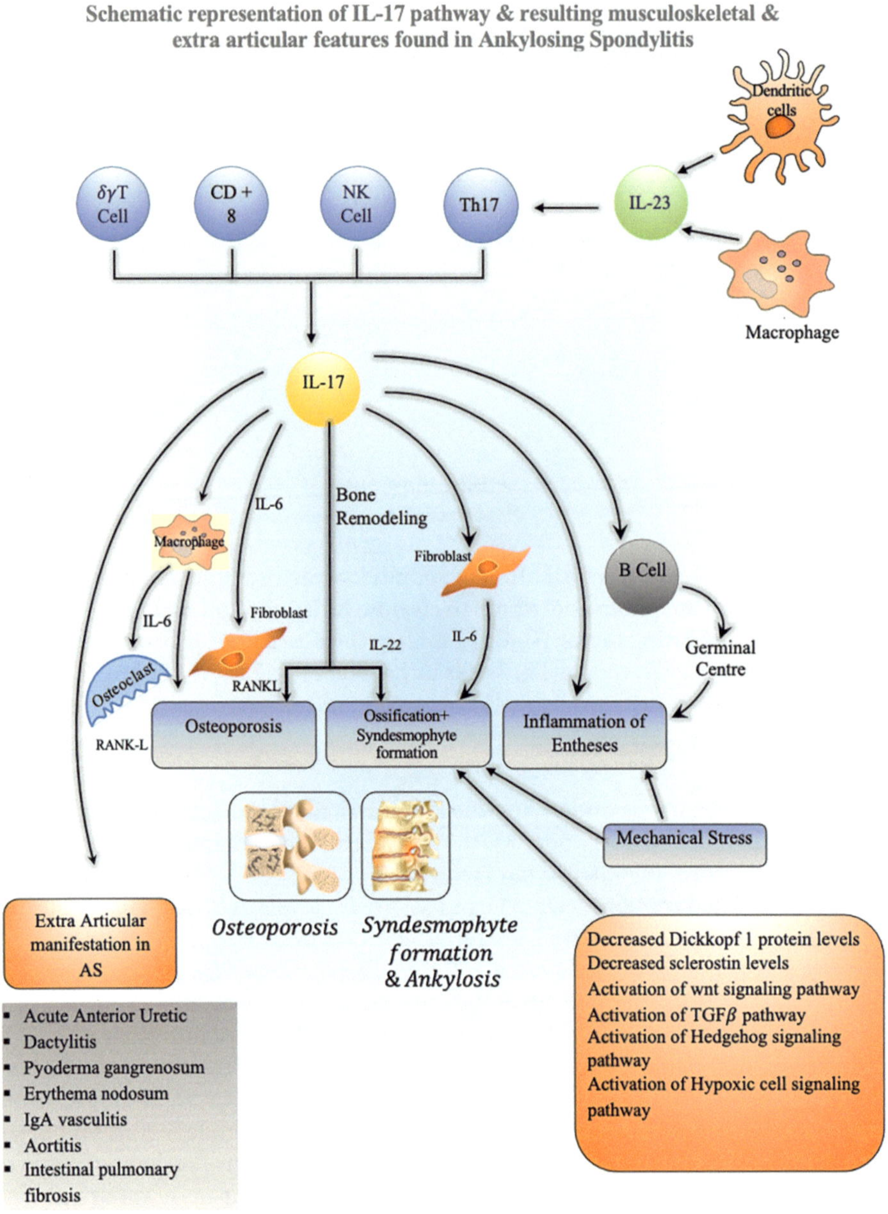

Figure 6.
Schematic representation of IL-17 pathway & resulting musculoskeletal & extra articular features found in ankylosing spondylitis.

This aberrant osteogenesis/proliferation leading to ankylosis occurs adjacent to and in connection to existing bone but extends beyond normal physiological boundaries, often along adjacent entheses [127].

There is MRI data in some patients demonstrating ossification where no previous inflammation has occurred in support of the theory that ossification occurs independently to chronic inflammation in AS [127].

MRI studies suggest active inflammatory lesions might evolve into 'remodelling' lesions characterised by mesenchymal tissue responses, ultimately leading to ossification [127]. Emerging literature suggests a range of processes resulting in heterotopic ossification of the tendons and ligaments (HOTL) [51]. HOTL is described as a dynamic process [51], similar to fracture repair, involving stages and a variety of signally pathways that start with inflammation, injury and trauma, followed by mesenchymal stromal cell recruitment, chondrocyte differentiation and finally ossification. More research is required to establish the role of HOTL in AS.

The rates and severity of bone formation vary significantly among AS patients [128].

Some studies have demonstrated patients with high markers of tissue turnover biomarkers experience more structural damage [127].

There are several pro inflammatory mediators involved in bone remodelling including tumour necrosis factor-α (TNF-α), insulin-like growth factor II (IGF-II), insulin-like growth factor-binding protein 5 (IGFBP5), prostaglandin reductase 1 (Ptgr1), latent-transforming growth factor beta-binding protein 3 (LTBP3), transforming growth factor beta-1 (TGF-β1), neutrophil elastase (NE), serum amyloid A-4 protein (SAA4), protein S100-A9 and prostaglandin-H2 D-isomerase [51].

Some researchers suggest cellular pyrophosphate exportation contributes to the pathological ossification during AS progression, which is regulated by pyrophosphate transfer-related genes, such as ANKH [128].

IL-17 impacts bone metabolism by activating the production of matrix metalloproteinases from macrophages [1]. IL-17 stimulates TNF-α production and can mediate osteoclast activation via shifting receptor activator of nuclear factor κB ligand (RANKL)/osteoprotegerin (OPG) balance towards RANKL. As OPG functions as a soluble receptor for RANKL, serving to neutralise RANKL and osteoclast formation, it is not surprising that low serum levels of OPG have been associated with osteopenia in AS [127].

IL-17A blockade may be more effective than TNF-α inhibition in halting pathological new bone formation [122, 129]. In fact, TNF-α inhibitors have been shown to accelerate ossification in some AS patients [122].

3.3 Extra-articular/musculoskeletal disease in AS

As with other areas in AS pathophysiology the exact mechanisms that are associated with the various systemic and organ specific manifestations of the disease remain unclear although HLA-B27 has been shown to be associated with acute anterior uveitis (AAU) [130]. However, one study reported that HLA-B27 negativity was associated with an increase in peripheral arthritis, dactylitis, and extra-articular manifestations including AAU [131].

One study demonstrated a relationship between HLA-B27 positivity in AS, aberrant IL-17 production can cause aortitis, acute anterior uveitis, and interstitial lung fibrosis [118]. Pathogen-associated molecular pattern (PAMP), damage-associated molecular pattern (DAMPS), natural cytotoxicity triggering receptor 2 (NPC2) and CD336 have been identified in extra-articular features of AS although more research is required to better qualifythe pathophysiology of these phenomena [118].

4. Conclusion

The pathogenesis and pathophysiology of Ankylosing Spondylitis (AS) is complex involving a variety of factors and interactions that remains to be fully understood. Genetic factors including a variety of HLA-B27 subset genes, ERAP 1, ERAP2, IL-23R and other genes are well documented in the literature, with novel genes and gene–gene interaction continuously identified in AS research. Dysregulation of the enteric microbiome with characteristic changes to certain bacterial, viral, fungal and interactions between microbiota are recognised in AS patients. There exists a corresponding aberrant immunological response with altered behaviour in DCs, macrophages, T cells, B cells that appear to be drive and be driven by the IL-17/IL-23 pathway. As such there is evidence that the pathophysiological response in AS is a combination of both autoinflammatory and autoimmune components, but further research is required to establish the intricate mechanisms involved. There remains controversy in the literature about mechanisms giving rise to the characteristic clinicical features of AS including sacroiliitis, spondylitis, ankylosis and whether these occur as a direct result of inflammation, or whether these arise independently as a result of altered mechanisms to bone metabolism in AS specifically.

The complete pathophyisiological pathways resulting in uveitis and other extra articular manifestations remain occult. Further research to establish complete understanding of factors involved in pathogenesis and pathophysiology of AS is required.

Acknowledgements

Thank you to IntechOpen for the opportunity to publish this chapter.

Conflict of interest

This author has no conflicts of interest to declare and has received no funding in writing this chapter.

Author details

Malini Alexander
University of South Wales, Pontypridd, UK

*Address all correspondence to: dr.alexander@rheumination.online

References

[1] Tsukazaki H, Kaito T. The role of the IL-23/IL-17 pathway in the athogenesis of spondyloarthritis. International Journal of Molecular Sciences. 2020;**21**(17):6401. DOI: 10.3390/ijms21176401

[2] Zhu W, He X, Cheng K, Zhang L, Chen D, Wang X, et al. Ankylosing spondylitis: Etiology, pathogenesis, and treatments. Bone Research. 2019;7:22. DOI: 10.1038/s41413-019-0057-8

[3] Tsui FW, Tsui HW, Akram A, Haroon N, Inman RD. The genetic basis of ankylosing spondylitis: New insights into disease pathogenesis. Application of Clinical Genetics. 2014;7:105-115. DOI: 10.2147/TACG.S37325

[4] Sehnal D, Bittrich S, Deshpande M, Svobodová R, Berka K, Bazgier V, et al. Mol* viewer: Modern web app for 3D visualization and analysis of large biomolecular structures. Nucleic Acids Research. 2001;**49**:W431-W437. DOI: 10.1093/nar/gkab314

[5] Berman HM, Westbrook J, Feng Z, Gilliland G, Bhat TN, Weissig H, et al. The protein data bank. Nucleic Acids Research. 2000;**28**:235-242

[6] Sharip A, Kunz J. Understanding the pathogenesis of spondyloarthritis. Biomolecules. 2020;**10**:1461. DOI: 10.3390/biom10101461

[7] Madden DR, Gorga JC, Strominger JL, Wiley DC. The structure of HLA-B27 reveals nonamer self-peptides bound in an extended conformation. Nature. 1991;**353**(6342):321-325

[8] Haridas V, Shetty P, Kumar MN, Vasanthakumar K, Haridas K, Khode V, et al. Human leukocyte antigen-B*27 allele subtype prevalence and disease association of ankylosing spondylitis among south Indian population. Indian Journal of Rheumatology. 2018;**13**:38-43. DOI: 10.4103/injr.injr_95_17

[9] Doğan HO, Şenol O, Karadağ A, Yıldız SN. Metabolomic profiling in ankylosing spondylitis using time-of-flight mass spectrometry. Clinical Nutrition ESPN. 2022;**50**:124-132. DOI: 10.1016/j.clnesp.2022.06.011

[10] Qin X, Zhu B, Jiang T, Tan J, Wu Z, Yuan Z, et al. miR-17-5p regulates heterotopic ossification by targeting ANKH in ankylosing spondylitis. Molecular Therapy-Nucleic Acids. 2019;**18**:696-707. DOI: 10.1016/j.omtn.2019.10.003

[11] Kim K, Bang SY, Lee S, Lee HS, Shim SC, Kang YM, et al. An HLA-C amino-acid variant in addition to HLA-B*27 confers risk for ankylosing spondylitis in the Korean population. Arthritis Research & Therapy. 2015;**17**:342. DOI: 10.1186/s13075-015-0855-3

[12] Nancy Z, Yan L, Hui S, Paul B, Liye C. From the genetics of ankylosing spondylitis to new biology and drug target discovery. Frontiers in Immunology. 2021;**12**:624632. DOI: 10.3389/fimmu.2021.624632

[13] Bowness P, Ridley A, Shaw J, Chan AT, Wong-Baeza I, Fleming M, et al. Th17 cells expressing KIR3DL2+ and responsive to HLA-B27 homodimers are increased in ankylosing spondylitis. Journal of Immunology. 2011;**186**(4):2672-2680. DOI: 10.4049/jimmunol.1002653

[14] Rysnik O, McHugh K, van Duivenvoorde L, van Tok M, Guggino G,

Taurog J, et al. Non-conventional forms of HLA-B27 are expressed in spondyloarthritis joints and gut tissue. Journal of Autoimmunity. 2016;**70**:12-21

[15] Breban M, Hill G. Chapter 8: Immune mechanisms: Adaptive immunity. In: Inman R, Sieper J, editors. The Oxford Textbook of Axial Spondyloarthritis. Oxford University Press; 2016

[16] Mauro D, Thomas R, Guggino G, Lories R, Brown MA, Ciccia F. Ankylosing spondylitis: An autoimmune or autoinflammatory disease? Nature Reviews Rheumatology. 2021;**17**:387-404. DOI: 10.1038/s41584-021-00625-y

[17] Brown MA, Edwards S, Hoyle E, Campbell S, Laval S, Daly AK, et al. Polymorphisms of the CYP2D6 gene increase susceptibility to ankylosing spondylitis. Human Molecular Genetics. 2000;**9**(11):1563-1566. DOI: 10.1093/hmg/9.11.1563

[18] Pimentel-Santos FM, Ligeiro D, Matos M, Mourão AF, Vieira de Sousa E, Pinto P, et al. ANKH and susceptibility to and severity of ankylosing spondylitis. The Journal of Rheumatology. 2012;**39**(1):131-134. DOI: 10.3899/jrheum.110681

[19] Evans DM, Spencer CC, Pointon JJ, Su Z, Harvey D, Kochan G, et al. Interaction between ERAP1 and HLA-B27 in ankylosing spondylitis implicates peptide handling in the mechanism for HLA-B27 in disease susceptibility. Nature Genetics. 2011;**43**(8):761-767. DOI: 10.1038/ng.873

[20] Costello ME, Ciccia F, Willner D, Warrington N, Robinson PC, Gardiner B, et al. Brief report: Intestinal dysbiosis in ankylosing spondylitis. Arthritis & Rheumatology. 2015;**67**(3):686-691. DOI: 10.1002/art.38967

[21] Chen B, Huang K, Ye L, Li Y, Zhang J, Zhang J, et al. Interleukin-37 is increased in ankylosing spondylitis patients and associated with disease activity. Journal of Translational Medicine. 2015;**13**(1):36. DOI: 10.1186/s12967-015-0394-3

[22] Rezaiemanesh A, Abdolmaleki M, Abdolmohammadi K, Aghaei H, Pakdel FD, Fatahi Y, et al. Immune cells involved in the pathogenesis of ankylosing spondylitis. Biomedicine & Pharmacotherapy. 2018;**100**:198-204. DOI: 10.1016/j.biopha.2018.01.108

[23] Stockwin LH, McGonagle D, Martin IG, Blair GE. Dendritic cells: Immunological sentinels with a central role in health and disease. Immunology & Cell Biology. 2000;**78**(2):91-102. DOI: 10.1046/j.1440-1711.2000.00888.x

[24] Wright PB, McEntegart A, McCarey D, McInnes IB, Siebert S, Milling SW. Ankylosing spondylitis patients display altered dendritic cell and T cell populations that implicate pathogenic roles for the IL-23 cytokine axis and intestinal inflammation. Rheumatology (Oxford, England). 2016;**55**(1):120-132. DOI: 10.1093/rheumatology/kev245

[25] Quaden DH, De Winter LM, Somers V. Detection of novel diagnostic antibodies in ankylosing spondylitis: An overview. Autoimmunity Reviews. 2016;**15**(8):820-832. DOI: 10.1016/j.autrev.2016.06.001

[26] Wilbrink R, Spoorenberg A, Verstappen GMPJ, Kroese FGM. B cell involvement in the pathogenesis of ankylosing spondylitis. International Journal of Molecular Sciences. 2021;**22**(24):13325. DOI: 10.3390/ijms222413325

[27] Hu Q, Sun Y, Li Y, Shi H, Teng J, Liu H, et al. Anti-SIRT1 autoantibody

is elevated in ankylosing spondylitis: A potential disease biomarker. BMC Immunology. 2018;**19**(1):38

[28] Guglielmi V, Vattemi G, Cecconi D, Fracasso G, Marini M, Tomelleri G. Acute sarcomeric m-line disease associated with ATP synthase subunit α autoantibodies in ankylosing spondylitis. Journal of Neuropathology & Experimental Neurology. 2018;**11**:987-992

[29] Fielder M, Pirt SJ, Tarpey I, Wilson C, Cunningham P, Ettelaie C, et al. Molecular mimicry and ankylosing spondylitis: Possible role of a novel sequence in pullulanase of *Klebsiella pneumoniae*. FEBS Letters. 1995;**369**(2-3):243-248. DOI: 10.1016/0014-5793(95)00760-7

[30] Stoll ML. Interactions of the innate and adaptive arms of the immune system in the pathogenesis of spondyloarthritis. Clinical and Experimental Rheumatology. 2011;**29**(2):322-330

[31] Ciccia F, Guggino G, Rizzo A, Saieva L, Peralta S, Giardina A, et al. Type 3 innate lymphoid cells producing IL-17 and IL-22 are expanded in the gut, in the peripheral blood, synovial fluid and bone marrow of patients with ankylosing spondylitis. Annals of the Rheumatic Diseases. 2015;**74**(9):1739-1747. DOI: 10.1136/annrheumdis-2014-206323

[32] Reinhardt A, Prinz I. Whodunit? The contribution of interleukin (IL)-17/IL-22-producing γδ T cells, αβ T cells, and innate lymphoid cells to the pathogenesis of spondyloarthritis. Frontiers in Immunology. 2018;**9**:885. DOI: 10.3389/fimmu.2018.00885

[33] Nie J, Li YY, Zheng SG, Tsun A, Li B. FOXP3(+) Treg cells and gender bias in autoimmune diseases. Frontiers in Immunology. 2015;**6**:493. DOI: 10.3389/fimmu.2015.00493

[34] Toussirot É, Laheurte C, Gaugler B, Gabriel D, Saas P. Increased IL-22- and IL-17A-producing mucosal-associated invariant T cells in the peripheral blood of patients with ankylosing spondylitis. Frontiers in Immunology. 2018;**9**:1610. DOI: 10.3389/fimmu.2018.01610

[35] Stebbings SM, Roberts RL. The interplay of genes with the gut microbiota in the aetiopathogenesis of spondyloarthropathies and Crohn's disease: Implications for future therapeutic targets. EMJ. Rheumatology. 2021;**8**(1):140-151. DOI: 10.33590/emjrheumatol/21-00025

[36] Gill T, Rosenbaum JT. Putative pathobionts in HLA-B27-associated spondyloarthropathy. Frontiers in Immunology. 2021;**11**:586494. DOI: 10.3389/fimmu.2020.586494

[37] Ley R, Lozupone C, Hamady M, Knight R, Gordon J. Worlds within worlds: Evolution of the vertebrate gut microbiota. Nature Reviews Microbiology. 2008;**6**:776-788. DOI: 10.1038/nrmicro1978

[38] Gill T, Asquith M, Rosenbaum JT, Colbert RA. The intestinal microbiome in spondyloarthritis. Current Opinion in Rheumatology. 2015;**27**(4):319-325. DOI: 10.1097/BOR.0000000000000187

[39] Schinocca C, Rizzo C, Fasano S, Grasso G, La Barbera L, Ciccia F, et al. Role of the IL-23/IL-17 pathway in rheumatic diseases: An overview. Frontiers in Immunology. 2021;**12**:637829. DOI: 10.3389/fimmu.2021.637829

[40] Harkins P, Burke E, Swales C, Silman A. 'All disease begins in the gut'—The role of the intestinal microbiome in ankylosing spondylitis. Rheumatology advances. Practice. 2021;**5**(3):rkab063. DOI: 10.1093/rap/rkab063

[41] Chukkapalli S, Kweh M, Gehlot P, Velsko I, Bhattacharyya I, Calise SJ, et al. Periodontal bacterial colonization in synovial tissues exacerbates collagen-induced arthritis in B10.RIII mice. Arthritis Research & Therapy. 2016;**18**:1, 161. DOI: 10.1186/s13075-016-1056-4

[42] Mielants H, De Keyser F, Baeten D, Van den Bosch F. Gut inflammation in the spondyloarthropathies. Current Rheumatology Reports. 2005;**7**(3):188-194. DOI: 10.1007/s11926-996-0038-y

[43] Bjarnason I, Helgason KO, Geirsson AJ, Sigthorsson G, Reynisdottir I, Gudbjartsson D, et al. Subclinical intestinal inflammation and sacroiliac changes in relatives of patients with ankylosing spondylitis. Gastroenterology. 2003;**125**(6):1598-1605. DOI: 10.1053/j.gastro.2003.08.035

[44] Tito RY, Cypers H, Joossens M, Varkas G, Van Praet L, Glorieus E, et al. Brief report: Dialister as a microbial marker of disease activity in Spondyloarthritis. Arthritis & Rheumatology. 2017;**69**(1):114-121. DOI: 10.1002/art.39802

[45] Wen C, Zheng Z, Shao T, Liu L, Xie Z, Le Chatelier E, et al. Quantitative metagenomics reveals unique gut microbiome biomarkers in ankylosing spondylitis. Genome Biology. 2017;**18**(1):142. DOI: 10.1186/s13059-017-1271-6

[46] Viladomiu M, Kivolowitz C, Abdulhamid A, Dogan B, Victorio D, Castellanos JG, et al. IgA-coated E. coli enriched in Crohn's disease spondyloarthritis promote TH17-dependent inflammation. Science Translational Medicine. 2017;**9**:aaf9655. DOI: 10.1126/scitranslmed.aaf9655

[47] Rodrigues IK, Andrigueti M, de Oliveira Gil ID, de Lucca SL, de Andrade KR, Pereira IA, et al. An investigation into the relationship between anti-helicobacter pylori and anti-Saccharomyces cerevisiae antibodies in patients with axial spondyloarthritis and Crohn disease. Rheumatology International. 2015;**35**(2):359-366. DOI: 10.1007/s00296-014-3088-x

[48] Manasson J, Wallach DS, Guggino G, Stapylton M, Badri MH, Solomon G, et al. Interleukin-17 inhibition in spondyloarthritis is associated with subclinical gut microbiome perturbations and a distinctive interleukin-25-driven intestinal inflammation. Arthritis & Rheumatology. 2020;**72**(4):645-657. DOI: 10.1002/art.41169

[49] Liu NN, Jiao N, Tan JC, Wang Z, Wu D, Wang AJ, et al. Multi-kingdom microbiota analyses identify bacterial-fungal interactions and biomarkers of colorectal cancer across cohorts. Nature Microbiology. 2022;**7**(2):238-250. DOI: 10.1038/s41564-021-01030-7

[50] Tomofuji Y, Kishikawa T, Maeda Y, Ogawa K, Nii T, Okuno T, et al. Whole gut virome analysis of 476 Japanese revealed a link between phage and autoimmune disease. Annals of the Rheumatic Diseases. 2022;**81**:278-288

[51] Zhang Q, Zhou D, Wang H, Tan J. Heterotopic ossification of tendon and ligament. Journal of Cellular and Molecular Medicine. 2020;**24**(10):5428-5437. DOI: 10.1111/jcmm.15240

[52] Inman R, Sieper J, editors. The Oxford Textbook of Axial Spondyloarthritis. Oxford University Press; 2016

[53] Brown M, Revielle J. Chapter 5: Genetics of Spondyloarthritis. In: Inman R, Sieper J, editors. The Oxford Textbook of Axial Spondyloarthritis. Oxford University Press; 2016

[54] Colbert R, Bowness P. Chapter 6: Immune Mechanisms: HLAB27. In: Inman R, Sieper J, editors. The Oxford Textbook of Axial Spondyloarthritis. Oxford University Press; 2016

[55] Bowness P. HLA B27 in health and disease: A double-edged sword? Rheumatology (Oxford). 2002;**41**:857-868

[56] Tavasolian F, Rashidi M, Hatam GR, Jeddi M, Hosseini AZ, Mosawi SH, et al. HLA, immune response, and susceptibility to COVID-19. Frontiers in Immunology. 2021;**11**:601886. DOI: 10.3389/fimmu.2020.601886

[57] Pereira A, Murtaza F, Kaplan AJ, Yan P. Initial anterior uveitis event associated with recent novel SARS-CoV-2 (COVID-19) infection in the setting of HLA-B27. American Journal of Ophthalmology Case Reports. 2022;**26**:101565. DOI: 10.1016/j.ajoc.2022.101565

[58] Apaydin H, Guven SC, Kucuksahin O, Omma A, Erten S. A case of human leukocyte antigen B27 positive reactive arthritis associated with severe acute respiratory syndrome coronavirus 2 infection. Northern Clinicals of Istanbul. 2021;**8**(4):423-424. DOI: 10.14744/nci.2020.88965

[59] Migliorini F, Torsiello E, Spiezia F, Oliva F, Tingart M, Maffulli N. Association between HLA genotypes and COVID-19 susceptibility, severity and progression: A comprehensive review of the literature. European Journal of Medical Research. 2021;**26**:84. DOI: 10.1186/s40001-021-00563-1

[60] Rizzo C, Camarda F, Donzella D, La Barbera L, Guggino G. Metabolomics: An emerging approach to understand pathogenesis and to assess diagnosis and response to treatment in spondyloarthritis. Cell. 2022;**11**(3):549. DOI: 10.3390/cells11030549

[61] Berlinberg AJ, Regner EH, Stahly A, Brar A, Reisz JA, Gerich ME, et al. Multi 'omics analysis of intestinal tissue in ankylosing spondylitis identifies alterations in the tryptophan metabolism pathway. Frontiers in Immunology. 2021;**12**:587119

[62] Ou J, Xiao M, Huang Y, Tu L, Chen Z, Cao S, et al. Serum metabolomics signatures associated with ankylosing spondylitis and TNF inhibitor therapy. Frontiers in Immunology. 2021;**12**:630791. DOI: 10.3389/fimmu.2021.630791

[63] Fischer R, Trudgian DC, Wright C, Thomas G, Bradbury LA, Brown MA, et al. Discovery of candidate serum proteomic and metabolomic biomarkers in ankylosing spondylitis. Molecular & Cellular Proteomics. 2012;**11**(2):M111.013904. DOI: 10.1074/mcp.M111.013904

[64] Rusman T, van Vollenhoven RF, van der Horst-Bruinsma IE. Gender differences in axial Spondyloarthritis: Women are not so lucky. Current Rheumatology Reports. 2018;**20**(6):35. DOI: 10.1007/s11926-018-0744-2

[65] Jo S, Lee EJ, Nam B, Kang J, Lee S, Youn J, et al. Effects of dihydrotestosterone on osteoblast activity in curdlan-administered SKG mice and osteoprogenitor cells in patients with ankylosing spondylitis. Arthritis Research & Therapy. 2020;**22**(1):121. DOI: 10.1186/s13075-020-02217-9

[66] Odeh S, Odeh M, Slobodin G, Shechner C, Saiegh L. Spinal SYNDESMOPHYTE score does not correlate with serum testosterone level IN male patients with

ankylosing spondylitis. Harefuah. 2019;**158**(9):568-570

[67] Gooren LJ, Giltay EJ, van Schaardenburg D, Dijkmans BA. Gonadal and adrenal sex steroids in ankylosing spondylitis. Rheumatic Disease Clinics of North America. 2000;**26**(4):969-987. DOI: 10.1016/s0889-857x(05)70179-4

[68] Traish A, Bolanos J, Nair S, Saad F, Morgentaler A. Do androgens modulate the pathophysiological pathways of inflammation? Appraising the contemporary evidence. J Clinical Medicine. 2018;**7**(12):549. DOI: 10.3390/jcm7120549

[69] Rusman T, van Bentum RE, van der Horst-Bruinsma IE. Sex and gender differences in axial spondyloarthritis: Myths and truths. Rheumatology (Oxford, England). 2020;**59**(Suppl. 4):iv38-iv46. DOI: 10.1093/rheumatology/keaa543

[70] James WH. Sex ratios and hormones in HLA related rheumatic diseases. Annals of Rheumatic Disease. 1991;**50**(6):401-404. DOI: 10.1136/ard.50.6.401

[71] Jeong H, Bae EK, Kim H, Eun YH, Kim IY, Kim H, et al. Estrogen attenuates the spondyloarthritis manifestations of the SKG arthritis model. Arthritis Research & Therapy. 2017;**19**(1):198. DOI: 10.1186/s13075-017-1407-9

[72] Bertoldo E, Adami G, Rossini M, Giollo A, Orsolini G, Viapiana O, et al. The emerging roles of endocrine hormones in different arthritic disorders. Frontiers in Endocrinology (Lausanne). 2021;**12**:620920. DOI: 10.3389/fendo.2021.620920

[73] Jeong H, Kim IY, Bae EK, Jeon CH, Ahn KS, Cha HS. Selective estrogen receptor modulator lasofoxifene suppresses spondyloarthritis manifestation and affects characteristics of gut microbiota in zymosan-induced SKG mice. Scientific Reports. 2021;**11**(1):11923. DOI: 10.1038/s41598-021-91320-1

[74] Edens C, Antonelli M. Polycystic ovarian syndrome in rheumatic disease [abstract]. Arthritis & Rheumatology. 2017;**69**(suppl. 10)

[75] Sharmeen S, Nomani H, Taub E, Carlson H, Yao Q. Polycystic ovary syndrome: Epidemiologic assessment of prevalence of systemic rheumatic and autoimmune diseases. Clinical Rheumatology. 2021;**40**(12):4837-4843. DOI: 10.1007/s10067-021-05850-0

[76] James W. Might HLA-B27 related diseases benefit from antiandrogenic treatment? Annals of Rheumatic Disease. 1995;**54**(6):531-532. DOI: 10.1136/ard.54.6.531

[77] Genre F, López-Mejías R, Miranda-Filloy JA, Ubilla B, Carnero-López B, Blanco R, et al. Adipokines, biomarkers of endothelial activation, and metabolic syndrome in patients with ankylosing spondylitis. Biomed Research International. 2014;**2014**:860651. DOI: 10.1155/2014/860651

[78] Liu M, Huang Y, Huang Z, Huang Q, Guo X, Wang Y, et al. Prevalence of metabolic syndrome and its associated factors in Chinese patients with ankylosing spondylitis. Diabetes Metab Syndr Obes. 2019;**12**:477-484. DOI: 10.2147/DMSO.S197745

[79] Petcharat C, Srinonprasert V, Chiowchanwisawakit P. Association between syndesmophyte and metabolic syndrome in patients with

psoriatic arthritis or ankylosing spondylitis: A cross-sectional study. BMC Musculoskeletal Disorders. 2021;**22**(1):367. DOI: 10.1186/s12891-021-04222-8

[80] Aradoini N, Talbi S, Mansouri S, et al. SAT0260 prevalence of metabolic syndrome in patients with ankylosing spondylitis in Morocco: A cross-sectional study of 103 cases. Annals of the Rheumatic Diseases. 2015;**74**:752-753

[81] Klein S, Flanagan K. Sex differences in immune responses. Nature Reviews in Immunology. 2016;**16**(10):626-638. DOI: 10.1038/nri.2016.90

[82] Macfarlane TV, Abbood HM, Pathan E, Gordon K, Hinz J, Macfarlane GJ. Relationship between diet and ankylosing spondylitis: A systematic review. European Journal of Rheumatology. 2018;**5**(1):45-52. DOI: 10.5152/eurjrheum.2017.16103

[83] Rashid T, Wilson C, Ebringer A. Raised incidence of ankylosing spondylitis among Inuit populations could be due to high HLA-B27 association and starch consumption. Rheumatology International. 2015;**35**(6):945-951. DOI: 10.1007/s00296-014-3164-2

[84] Popa SL, Dumitrascu DI, Brata VD, Duse TA, Florea MD, Ismaiel A, et al. Nutrition in spondyloarthritis and related immune-mediated disorders. Nutrients. 2022;**14**(6):1278. DOI: 10.3390/nu14061278

[85] Montoya J, Matta NB, Suchon P, Guzian MC, Lambert NC, Mattei JP, et al. Patients with ankylosing spondylitis have been breast fed less often than healthy controls: A case-control retrospective study. Annals of the Rheumatic Diseases. 2016;**75**(5):879-882. DOI: 10.1136/annrheumdis-2015-208187

[86] Voruganti A, Bowness P. New developments in our understanding of ankylosing spondylitis pathogenesis. Immunology. 2020;**161**(2):94-102. DOI: 10.1111/imm.13242

[87] Akar S, Kaplan YC, Ecemiş S, Keskin-Arslan E, Gercik Ö, Gücenmez S, et al. The role of smoking in the development and progression of structural damage in axial SpA patients: A systematic review and meta-analysis. European Journal of Rheumatology. 2018;**6**(4):184-192. DOI: 10.5152/eurjrheum.2019.19073

[88] Farouk HM, Abdel-Rahman MA, Hassan RM. Relationship between smoking, clinical, inflammatory, and radiographic parameters in patients with ankylosing spondylitis. Egyptian Rheumatology and Rehabilitation. 2021;**48**:26. DOI: 10.1186/s43166-021-00076-z

[89] Min HK, Lee J, Ju JH, Park SH, Kwok SK. Alcohol consumption as a predictor of the progression of spinal structural damage in axial spondyloarthritis: Data from the Catholic axial Spondyloarthritis cohort (CASCO). Arthritis Research & Therapy. 2019;**21**:187. DOI: 10.1186/s13075-019-1970-3

[90] Shiue I. Relationship of environmental exposures and ankylosing spondylitis and spinal mobility: US National Health and nutrition examination survey, 2009-2010. International Journal of Environmental Health Research. 2015;**25**:322-329. DOI: 10.1080/09603123.2014.945512

[91] Vojdani A, Pollard KM, Campbell AW. Environmental triggers and autoimmunity. Autoimmune Diseases. 2014;**2014**:798029. DOI: 10.1155/2014/798029

[92] Kharrazian D. Exposure to environmental toxins and autoimmune

eonditions. Integrative Medicine (Encinitas). 2021;**20**(2):20-24

[93] Khan MF, Wang H. Environmental exposures and autoimmune diseases: Contribution of gut microbiome. Frontiers in Immunology. 2020;**10**(10):3094. DOI: 10.3389/fimmu.2019.03094

[94] Bay-Jensen AC, Wichuk S, Byrjalsen I, Leeming DJ, Morency N, Christiansen C, et al. Circulating protein fragments of cartilage and connective tissue degradation are diagnostic and prognostic markers of rheumatoid arthritis and ankylosing spondylitis. PLoS One. 2013;**8**(1):e54504. DOI: 10.1371/journal.pone.0054504

[95] Chelakkot C, Ghim J, Ryu SH. Mechanisms regulating intestinal barrier integrity and its pathological implications. Experimental & Molecular Medicine. 2018;**50**:1-9. DOI: 10.1038/s12276-018-0126-x

[96] Rodgers KR, Gui J, Dinulos MB, Chou RC. Ehlers-Danlos syndrome hypermobility type is associated with rheumatic diseases. Scientific Reports. 2017;**7**:39636. DOI: 10.1038/srep39636

[97] Nallegowda M, Singh U, Khanna M, Kumar R. Coexistence of ankylosing spondylosis with benign joint hypermobility syndrome. Are they complementary to each other? Indian Journal of Physical Medicine and Rehabilitation. 2007;**18**:15-20

[98] Ognenovski V, Stewart S. AB0567 coexistence of spondyloarthropathy and hypermobility joint syndrome: A report of seven cases. Annals of the Rheumatic Diseases. 2013;**72**:A962-A963

[99] Nallegowda M, Singh U, Khanna M, Kumar R. Coexistence of ankylosing spondylosis with benign joint hypermobility syndrome. Are they complementary to each other? Indian Journal of Physical Medicine and Rehabilitation. 2001

[100] Shur NF, Shur JD, Rennie WJ, Moorthy A. Concurrent joint hypermobility syndrome and spondyloarthropathy: A new spondyloarthropathy subgroup with a less severe disease phenotype? Journal of Clinical Rheumatology. 2020;**26**(3):99-103. DOI: 10.1097/RHU.0000000000000959

[101] Viitanen JV. Do pathological opposites cancel each other out? Do all patients with both hypermobility and spondylarthropathy fulfill a criterion of any disease? Scandinavian Journal of Rheumatology. 1999;**28**(2):120-122. DOI: 10.1080/030097499442603

[102] Roberts RL, Wallace MC, Jones GT, van Rij AM, Merriman TR, Harrison A, et al. Prevalence of HLA-B27 in the New Zealand population: Effect of age and ethnicity. Arthritis Research & Therapy. 2013;**15**(5):R158. DOI: 10.1186/ar4341

[103] Khan MA. Race-related differences in HLA association with ankylosing spondylitis and Reiter's disease in American blacks and whites. Journal of the National Medical Association. 1978;**70**(1):41-42

[104] Jamalyaria F, Ward MM, Assassi S, Learch TJ, Lee M, Gensler LS, et al. Ethnicity and disease severity in ankylosing spondylitis a cross-sectional analysis of three ethnic groups. Clinical Rheumatology. 2017;**36**(10):2359-2364. DOI: 10.1007/s10067-017-3767-6

[105] Muñoz-Villanueva MC, Muñoz-GomarizE,Escudero-ContrerasA, Pèrez-Guijo V, Collantes-Estévez E. Biological and clinical markers of disease

activity in ankylosing spondylitis. The Journal of Rheumatology. 2003;**30**(12):2729-2732

[106] Meri S, Partanen J, Leirisalo-Repo M, Repo H. Complement activation and HLA-B27. Annals of the Rheumatic Diseases. 1988;**47**(3):210-214. DOI: 10.1136/ard.47.3.210

[107] Yang C, Ding P, Wang Q, Zhang L, Zhang X, Zhao J, et al. Inhibition of complement retards ankylosing spondylitis progression. Scientific Reports. 2016;**6**:34643. DOI: 10.1038/srep34643

[108] Hokstad I, Deyab G, Fagerland MW, Lyberg T, Hjeltnes G, Førre Ø, et al. Tumor necrosis factor inhibitors are associated with reduced complement activation in spondylarthropathies: An observational study. PLoS One. 2019;**14**(7):e0220079. DOI: 10.1371/journal.pone.0220079

[109] Jørgensen CM, Troldborg A, Hansen AG, Thiel S, Jurik AG, Kiil RM, et al. POS0059 complement proteins are elevated in patients with axSpA compared with relevant controls of patients with low back pain and spa-features without axSpA. Annals of the Rheumatic Diseases. 2022;**81**(Suppl. 1):245. DOI: 10.1136/annrheumdis-2022-eular.3846

[110] Kinsella TD, Vasey EL, FB. Serum complement and immunoglobulin levels in sporadic and familial ankylosing spondylitis. The Journal of Rheumatology. 1975;**2**:308-313

[111] Krauledat PB, Krapf FE, Manger B. Kalden JR. Evaluation of plasma C3d and immune complex determinations in the assessment of disease activity of patients with rheumatoid arthritis, systemic lupus erythematosus, and spondylitis ancylopoetica. Rheumatology International. 1985;**5**:97-101

[112] Panayi GS, Slaney J, Williams BD. Circulating immune complexes in patients with ankylosing spondylitis. Annals of the Rheumatic Diseases. 1980;**39**:445-448

[113] Aydin SZ, Atagunduz P, Inanc N, Bicakcigil M, Tasan D, Temel M, et al. Mannose binding lectin levels in spondyloarthropathies. The Journal of Rheumatology. 2007;**34**(10):2075-2077

[114] Colbert RA, DeLay ML, Layh-Schmitt G, Sowders DP. HLA-B27 misfolding and spondyloarthropathies. Adv. Exp. Med. Biol. 2009;**649**:217-234. DOI: 10.1007/978-1-4419-0298-6_16

[115] Noordenbos T, Baeten D. Chapter 7: Immune mechanisms: Innate immunity. In: Inman R, Sieper J, editors. The Oxford Textbook of Axial Spondyloarthritis. Oxford University Press; 2016

[116] Peruzzi M, Wagtmann N, Long EO. A p70 killer cell inhibitory receptor specific for several HLA-B allotypes discriminates among peptides bound to HLA-B*2705. Journal of Experimental Medicine. 1996;**184**:1585-1590

[117] Stewart-Jones GB, di Gleria K, Kollnberger S, McMichael AJ, Jones EY, Bowness P. Crystal structures and KIR3DL1 recognition of three immunodominant viral peptides complexed to HLA-B*2705. European Journal of Immunology. 2005;**35**(2):341-351

[118] Liao HT, Tsai CY, Lai CC, Hsieh SC, Sun YS, Li KJ, et al. The potential role of genetics, environmental factors, and gut dysbiosis in the aberrant non-coding RNA expression to mediate

inflammation and osteoclastogenic/osteogenic differentiation in ankylosing spondylitis. Frontiers in Cell and Developmental Biology. 2022;**9**:748063

[119] Russell T, Bridgewood C, Rowe H, Altaie A, Jones E, McGonagle D. Cytokine "fine tuning" of enthesis tissue homeostasis as a pointer to spondyloarthritis pathogenesis with a focus on relevant TNF and IL-17 targeted therapies. Seminars in Immunopathology. 2021;**43**(2):193-206

[120] Boyle LH, Goodall JC, Opat SS, Gaston JSH. The recognition of HLA-B27 by human CD4+ T lymphocytes. Journal of Immunology. 2001;**167**:2619-2624

[121] Rosenbaum JT, Davey MP. Time for a gut check: Evidence for the hypothesis that HLA-B27 predisposes to ankylosing spondylitis by altering the microbiome. Arthritis & Rheumatology. 2011;**63**(11):3195-3198. DOI: 10.1002/art.30558

[122] Baeten D, Adamopoulos IE. IL-23 inhibition in ankylosing spondylitis: Where did it go wrong? Frontiers in Immunology. 2021;**11**:623874. DOI: 10.3389/fimmu.2020.623874

[123] Wang M, Liu C, Bond A, Yang J, Zhou X, Wang J, et al. Dysfunction of regulatory T cells in patients with ankylosing spondylitis is associated with a loss of Tim-3. International Immunopharmacology. 2018;**59**:53-60. DOI: 10.1016/j.intimp.2018.03.032

[124] Yan J, Zhang Y, Zhang JP, Liang J, Li L, Zheng L. Tim-3 expression defines regulatory T cells in human tumors. PLoS One. 2013;**8**(3):e58006. DOI: 10.1371/journal.pone.0058006

[125] Lin S, Qiu M, Chen J. IL-4 modulates macrophage polarization in ankylosing spondylitis. Cellular Physiology and Biochemistry. 2015;**35**:2213-2222. DOI: 10.1159/000374026

[126] Rossini M, Viapiana O, Idolazzi L, Ghellere F, Fracassi E, Troplini S, et al. Higher level of dickkopf-1 is associated with low bone mineral density and higher prevalence of vertebral fractures in patients with ankylosing spondylitis. Calcified Tissue International. 2016;**98**:438-445. DOI: 10.1007/s00223-015-0093-3

[127] Lories BR, Schett G. Chapter 10: Patholog. In: Inman R, Sieper J, editors. The Oxford Textbook of Axial Spondyloarthritis. Oxford University Press; 2016

[128] Slobodin G, Rosner I, Odeh M. Bone formation in ankylosing spondylitis. OA Arthritis. 2013;**1**(1):7

[129] Braun J, Baraliakos X, Deodhar A, Baeten D, Sieper J, Emery P, et al. MEASURE 1 study group. Effect of secukinumab on clinical and radiographic outcomes in ankylosing spondylitis: 2-year results from the randomised phase III measure 1 study. Annals of the Rheumatic Diseases. 2017;**76**(6):1070-1077. DOI: 10.1136/annrheumdis-2016-209730

[130] Chang JH, McCluskey PJ, Wakefield D. Acute anterior uveitis and HLA-B27. Survey of Ophthalmology. 2005;**50**(4):364-388. DOI: 10.1016/j.survophthal.2005.04.003

[131] Arévalo M, Gratacós Masmitjà J, Moreno M, Calvet J, Orellana C, Ruiz D, et al. Influence of HLA-B27 on the ankylosing spondylitis phenotype: Results from the REGISPONSER database. Arthritis Research & Therapy. 2018;**20**(1):221. DOI: 10.1186/s13075-018-1724-7

Chapter 5

Treatment Modalities of Ankylosing Spondylitis

Rajeshwar Nath Srivastava, Shatakshi Pant, Sudeepti Ratan Srivastava, Amar Chandra Sharma and Saloni Raj

Abstract

Ankylosing spondylitis is a chronic inflammatory arthropathy of young adults which primarily affects the axial skeleton. The pathogenesis of AS is unclear, but it is thought to be caused by an early inflammatory phase followed by ossification that may induce local osteitis. It has also been linked to an increase in morbidity and mortality and is known to have a debilitating impact on QoL of the patients. Whereby, CRP and ESR are used for assessment of the disease activity and determination of treatment efficacy, HLA-B27 is considered the best biomarker for AS diagnosis. The conventional therapeutic regimen like NSAIDs and DMARDs alone are not effective in controlling symptoms and indicators of disease; however, when combined with the physical therapy, great improvement in the QoL of the patients has been observed. The outlook for AS has improved remarkably with the advent of biologics that blocks key inflammatory cytokines such as TNF inhibitors. Biologics aids in halting disease progression, and can be used concomitantly with other medications for pain management. In this chapter, barring surgical interventions, we will discuss about the non-pharmacological and pharmacological therapies routinely employed for the treatment of AS, as well as the novel therapeutics currently under study.

Keywords: ankylosing spondylitis, QoL, HLA-B27, NSAIDs, DMARDs

1. Introduction

Ankylosing spondylitis (AS) is defined as a persistent inflammatory autoimmune disorder, primarily affecting the axial skeleton; mostly joints of the spine, sacroiliac joints (SIJs), and their adjoining soft tissues. Patients with AS usually present with reduced spinal mobility and inflammatory low back pain (LBP). In AS, peripheral joint arthritis corresponds with the disease severity, but it is typically milder when compared to other seronegative spondyloarthropathies (SpA). Radiographic change in the form of sacroiliitis is one of the early sign of AS. In addition, cartilage thinning and bone condensation are also observed on both sides of the SIJs. Progression of this disease can lead to bony ankylosis of both SIJs and joints of the lumbar spine, also known as the "bamboo spine." There are instances where end-stage arthritis develops in the hip joints resulting in ankylosis, but it is uncommon at other sites. It is common to develop uveitis, and most cases can often be controlled with topical steroids [1–4].

AS is a member of the SpA category of rheumatic disease, i.e., diseases that present common genetic and clinical manifestations. It occurs predominantly in males and presents itself preferably in the early twenties and rarely after 45 years of age. It has been found to occur in 1 of every 200 people. AS is found to be more common in Europe (prevalence estimate of 23.8 per 10,000) followed by Asia (16.7 per 10,000). In India, the estimated diagnosed prevalence of AS is currently 1.65 million, and according to GlobalData's "Pharmaceutical Intelligence Center, " it is anticipated to rise annually by 2.95% from now until 2028 to reach 2.0 million [5–8]. The etiology of AS remains ambiguous to date, likewise other autoimmune disorders, AS is known to develop through a complex interplay of genetic and environmental factors. Studies have reported more than 100 gene loci to be in association with AS, but in sync, they account for only about 30% of AS heritability. A strong correlation of major histocompatibility antigen (MHC) class I allele HLA-B27 with AS has been established, thus HLA-B27 remains the best-known biomarker for the prognosis of AS, although only 1–2% population with HLA-B27 positive allele are known to develop AS. In addition, elevated levels of CRP and ESR are also detected in the serum of patients with AS [2, 4].

Treatment of patients with active AS involves improving functional ability, maintaining spinal flexibility, correct posture, and relieving symptoms. The conventional therapeutic regimen like Disease Modifying Anti Rheumatic Drugs (DMARDs) and Non Steroidal Anti Inflammatory Drugs (NSAIDs) are not really effective in controlling symptoms and indicators of disease, as well as in halting disease progression. However, with the advent of biologics that blocks key inflammatory cytokines such as Tumor Necrosis Factor (TNF), the outlook for AS has improved. In the short and medium-term, ongoing research has shown that these agents are effective and safe. Longer-term studies are also needed to determine whether these medicines are true disease modifiers in AS. In this chapter, we will discuss in-depth the treatment modalities currently employed and understudied for the treatment of AS [2, 4, 9].

2. Non-pharmacological treatment

There are numerous pharmacological and non-pharmacological treatments available to alleviate back and SIJ stiffness and pain while enhancing spinal and peripheral joint mobility. But, the long-term management of AS calls for a mix of medication, physical therapy, and psychosocial interventions. The main challenge is therefore to reduce the impact of AS on patients and the healthcare system. A key component of managing AS is supervised physical therapy, which has the potential to increase the efficacy of exercise regimens and result in a quicker and longer-lasting improvement in AS symptomatology [10].

2.1 Physical therapy

Physical therapy is listed as one of the non-pharmacological therapeutic strategy for the treatment of AS in contemporary, internationally accepted expert consensus documents because AS is an evolving condition. Physical therapy may include posture training, strengthening, flexibility or stretching and deep breathing exercises, which can be provided both individually and in groups. Even though many people with AS can benefit from exercise, not all programs are effective for everyone. Some people might benefit from gentle, low-impact exercises or those that concentrate on easing pain or stress [11, 12].

2.1.1 Strengthening, stretching and deep breathing exercises

The Spondylitis Association of America claims that developing stronger core muscles can help people with AS reduce back pain as well as pressure on their spines. The muscles that support the spine is known as core muscles, including the abdominal muscles. Stretching exercises such as spinal flexion can help the patient with AS in maintaining their mobility and reducing the risk of developing joint fusion. AS patients may experience breathing problems due to limited chest expansion. Therefore, physiotherapists may advise deep breathing exercises that aid in strengthening the diaphragm and increasing lung capacity [11].

2.1.2 Balneotherapy

Balneotherapy is a traditional physical therapy that involves spa treatment. Since ancient times, it has been used to treat rheumatic diseases. One physiological result of being exposed to heat during a spa treatment is increased blood circulation in the tissues. Heat exposure to inflamed tissues promotes the flow of fresh blood through the tissues and speeds up the removal of toxic elements, thereby promoting tissue healing [13].

2.1.3 Chiropractic therapy

The term "chiropractic" is used to describe a wide range of therapeutic modalities. These may combine manual therapies, passive modalities, exercise regimens, high-velocity spinal manipulation, no touch therapy, touch therapy, and pain education, but are not limited to those. The American College of Rheumatology, the Spondylitis Association of America, and Spartan published the "Treatment Guidelines in Axial Spondyloarthritis" in 2015, and they strongly advise against using high-velocity thrusts to manipulate the spine in AS patients who have spinal osteoporosis or spinal fusion. Axial spondyloarthritis patients should not undergo spinal manipulation due to the risk of undiagnosed osteoporosis and the potential side effects of manipulating joints that are actively inflamed. Prior to starting chiropractic treatment, extreme caution should be exercised [14].

Due to the risk of undiagnosed osteoporosis and the unknown effects of joint manipulation in actively inflamed joints, spinal manipulation in any patient with established axial spondyloarthritis should be avoided. Prior to starting chiropractic treatment, extreme caution should be taken. Spinal fractures, spinal cord damage, and even paraplegia are risks for people with axial spondyloarthritis [14].

2.2 Yoga

Yoga is a discipline involving mind–body practices. In both clinical and non-clinical populations, it promotes health benefits through physical postures, breathing techniques, relaxation techniques, and meditation. Yoga is known to improve various musculoskeletal problems such as back and neck pain, osteoarthritis, etc. Additionally, it has been effective in improving pain management and spinal flexibility in chronic low back pain patients. Researchers found that yoga practice can help reduce inflammation and improve the range of motion in musculoskeletal disorders by down-regulating the nuclear factor κ β (F-κβ) [15].

In a study, researchers validated a yoga module for the treatment of AS based on the improvements observed in the spinal flexibility and chronic pain. The module included amalgamation of different yoga practices such as loosening, breathing, asanas, pranayama and yogic cleansing techniques. It was concluded that following the module for at least 30 minutes every day for a minimum of 3 days a week for 3 months, can help AS patients in improving their quality of life (QoL). Moreover, the use of breathing exercises and relaxation techniques can potentially increase one's pain tolerance and sensitivity. Increased endorphin levels and decreased hypothalamus–pituitary–adrenal (HPA) axis activity are also found to be linked to yoga practice [16].

3. Pharmacological treatment

3.1 NSAIDs

NSAIDs are a broad class of medications with a wide range of structural and functional characteristics. Most of these are weak organic acids (comprising of an acidic moiety along with an aromatic functional group). NSAIDs can be broadly classified based on their chemical structure, Cyclooxygenase (COX)/prostaglandin-endoperoxide synthase (PGHS) inhibition, and bioavailability in the serum. NSAIDs primarily function by inhibiting the COX enzyme (COX-1 and COX-2), which converts arachidonic to prostaglandins (PGs), thereby mediating inflammation and pain. COX-1 exclusively produces PGs crucial for maintenance normal physiological functions (maintenance of endocrine and renal functions, integrity of gastric mucosa, and hemostasis). Under normal physiological conditions, COX-1 is found in higher concentrations in the platelets, vascular endothelial cells, the stomach, and kidney collecting tubules. On the contrary, COX-2 exclusively produces PGs that mediates local inflammation, and is almost undetectable in most of the tissues. Traditional NSAIDs are non-selective meaning they can inhibit both COX-1 and COX-2. The new class of NSAIDS that selectively inhibits COX-2 is known as COX inhibitors [17].

NSAIDs form the first line of treatment for patients with active AS because of their efficacy in reducing pain and inflammation. Phenylbutazone was the first most popular drug to be used for AS treatment, giving good results. However, drug tolerance to patients was poor, additionally causing hematological adverse events (severe agranulocytosis). Several clinical trials conducted to ascertain the effectiveness and safety of NSAIDs in subjects with active and stable AS were evaluated. Results from 9 out of 15 clinical trials showed that indomethacin, a COX inhibitor was associated with neurological adverse events (AEs) such as headache and dizziness. Moreover, indomethacin 50 mg slow release tablets were found to be equally effective to indomethacin 25 mg capsule, but the former had fewer side effects. In most of the subjects, piroxicam (traditional NSAID) and aceclofenac (COX inhibitor) were found to be better tolerated than indomethacin. Aceclofenac exhibits lower risk of developing cardiovascular, renal, and gastrointestinal side effects when compared to traditional NSAIDs, naproxen and diclofenac [18–20].

There are no preferred NSAIDs for treatment of AS, but it is conditionally recommended that NSAIDs can be used continuously in subjects with persistently active, symptomatic diseases, with doses adjusted according to the severity of the disease, patient preferences, and co-morbidities. Since, the side effects outweigh the benefit of continuous treatment with NSAIDs in delaying the radiographic progression of the disease. On-demand treatment is conditionally recommended for management of subjects with stable disease activity [20].

3.2 Analgesics, muscle relaxants and corticosteroids

In patients with poor tolerance to NSAIDs, adjuvant therapy can be given which includes analgesics, muscle relaxants, and corticosteroids. In patients with NSAID intolerance, analgesics such as paracetamol (acetaminophen) and dextropropoxyphene is given concomitantly with muscle relaxant like tetrazepam in order to reduce pain and stiffness. Not much data is available on the use of glucocorticoids for the management of AS. However use of low and moderate-dose corticosteroids orally, has not been found much effective in relieving AS symptoms. In recent RCTs (randomized controlled trials), pulse therapy using a high dose of corticosteroids both orally and intravenously has produced favorable results. It is advised that administration of corticosteroid injections should generally be restricted to no more than three times per year, with at least 3 months passing between each injection in the same joint [19–23].

3.3 DMARDs

DMARDs form the second line of treatment for patients with AS who do not show promising results with NSAIDs and analgesics. They are pharmaceutical agents that suppress autoimmune activity and slow down or stop joint degeneration in order to promote remission. Given that DMARDs are slow-acting medications with a delayed onset of between 6 weeks and 6 months, the treatment should be started as soon as possible because early implementation yields better outcomes [24].

There are different types of DMARDs such as Biologic DMARDs (bDMARDs), targeted synthetic DMARDs (tsDMARDs), and traditional synthetic DMARDs (csDMARDs). For patients with newly diagnosed rheumatoid arthritis (RA), csDMARDs are typically used as the first line of treatment. If first-line therapy is not tolerated or is ineffective, bDMARDs or tsDMARDs are advised [24].

csDMARDs such as Leflunomide (LEF), methotrexate (MTX), sulfasalazine (SSZ), and hydroxychloroquine (HCQ) are used more frequently than other agents with a lower efficacy and safety profile, which includes gold salts, azathioprine, d-penicillamine, cyclosporine, minocycline, etc. The mechanism of action of these medications results in a non-targeted immune system suppression [24].

3.3.1 Methotrexate

As an anti-metabolite, MTX inhibits dihydrofolate reductase (DHFR) through competitive inhibition, thereby preventing DNA synthesis. MTX has exhibited promising results in the treatment of RA, but in AS not much evidence is available on the efficacy of the drug. MTX is rarely used for AS treatment but is prescribed to AS patients who show intolerance to SZZ [25].

3.3.2 Sulfasalazine

Following its initial development and use in RA, SSZ showed promise in the treatment of inflammatory bowel disease. Salicylic acid and the antibacterial compound sulfapyridine are combined to form SSZ. SSZ is normally prescribed in the dosage of 500 or 1000 mg twice a day. The rationale for using SSZ in AS stems from the description of inflammatory lesions in the ileum of AS patients, as well as the frequent correlation between AS and inflammatory bowel disease (IBD). In addition, it has been proposed that intestinal bacteria may cause AS (such as *Klebsiella pneumoniae*). As a result, SSZ has been investigated as a potential therapeutic option for AS patients [19].

In another study conducted, SSZ did not prove to be effective in the management of AS in terms of reducing pain, disease activity, radiographic progression, or enhancing physical function and spinal mobility. Contrary, SSZ has exhibited statistically significant benefits in lowering the ESR and reducing spinal stiffness. The effect size, however, was extremely small and not clinically significant. Moreover, it was observed that withdrawal due to side effects was more common in patients with AS treated with SSZ [26].

SSZ or MTX are conditionally recommended in patients who have prominent peripheral manifestations (such as peripheral arthritis) with few or no axial skeleton symptoms or when TNFi are not available or patients exhibiting contraindications to TNFi. In patients with contraindications to TNFi due to tuberculosis, other chronic infections, or high risk of recurrent infections, SSZ is preferred over secukinumab, ixekizumab and tofacitinib [20].

3.4 Bisphosphonates

Bisphosphonates are stable chemical derivatives of naturally occurring inorganic pyrophosphates (PPi). The PPi is formed by the esterification of two phosphate groups. Bisphosphonates act by promoting apoptosis of osteoclasts, thus they have become the primary therapy for the treatment of skeletal conditions marked by increased osteoclast-mediated bone resorption [27]. Among the conditions commonly treated with bisphosphonates are Paget's disease, hypercalcemia, osteoporosis and malignant bone diseases. Furthermore, bisphosphonates have anti-inflammatory properties, which may explain their use in treating inflammatory rheumatic diseases like AS [28].

Studies have reported positive results in the treatment of AS with pamidronate, as it successfully treated both spinal and peripheral disease, enthesitis included, when applied intravenously. Clinical improvements, in general, were found to be mild and delayed, but they did not correlate with the laboratory parameters of inflammation. Alternatively, pamidronate favored bone turnover by reducing markers of bone resorption and formation. Another study involving a comparison of infliximab, it was exhibited that short-term therapy for AS with neridronate is effective. Thus, for long-term treatment of AS, bisphosphonates alone or in combination with anti-TNF may be considered. It was observed that turnover of subchondral bone is reduced by bisphosphonates, which also have anti-inflammatory effects turnover [28–30].

3.5 Thalidomides

An analogue of racemic glutamic acid, thalidomide is composed of the S(−) and R(+) enantiomers, which interconvert under physiological circumstances. The R(+) form appears to act as a sedative, likely via sleep receptors in the forebrain, whereas the S(−) form potently inhibits the release of tumor necrosis factor (TNF) from peripheral mononuclear blood cells [30]. Since the 1990s, thalidomide has been used to treat AS in China, where it has been proven to be both effective and safe over the long term. Strict adherence to the System for Thalidomide Education and Prescription Safety (STEPS) programme is undertaken while prescribing this medication, because of the drug's toxicity to the developing fetus. Thereby explaining why the thalidomide rates are significantly lower in patients with shorter disease duration [31, 32].

3.6 Cytokine therapy

3.6.1 Tumor necrosis factor inhibitors

The development of TNF inhibitors (TNFi) has been the most significant advancement in the management of AS in recent years. These are referred to as biologics chiefly targeting the inflammatory modulators that are known to play important role in disease pathogenesis. TNFi in the treatment of AS mainly focuses on TNF-alpha (TNF-α) inhibition. TNF-α is known to play a central role in the inflammation of the axial skeleton and entheses in AS patients. It can activate various signaling pathways, thereby mediating the release of various inflammatory mediators like interleukins (ILs), and the activation of immune cells such as T cells, B-cells, or macrophages. TNFi is given to patients who exhibit intolerance to NSAIDs and analgesics and administered subcutaneously with infliximab as an exception, which is given through infusion [32–36]. A systematic review demonstrated that after etanercept [(1.2% of the patients producing anti-drug antibodies (ADAs)], golimumab was the least immunogenic (3.8%) of the TNFi, followed by infliximab (25.3%), adalimumab (14.1%), and certolizumab (6.9%) [37].

TNFi is strongly recommended to patients with active disease exhibiting no response or contraindications to at least two different NSAIDs therapy for over a month. There is no preferred choice of TNFi for the treatment of AS. In case of patients showing secondary non-response to the first TNFi used for treatment, switching to another TNFi is conditionally recommended. In patients with recurring uveitis or inflammatory bowel disease (IBD) use of monoclonal TNFi is recommended. Patients with stable disease activity being treated with combination of NSAID and TNFi, discontinuation of NSAID and treatment of TNFi alone is recommended [20].

3.6.1.1 Etanercept

Etanercept (ETN) is a TNF-α binding and TNF-α inactivating dimeric fusion protein composed of the human p75 TNF receptor and the Fc region of human Immunoglobulin G1 (IgG1). Unlike adalimumab (ADA) and IFX, it also binds to lymphotoxin-α [33]. ETN neutralizes this fusion protein, which is highly compatible with soluble TNF-α in plasma and on the surface of cell membranes, resulting in loss of the biological activity of TNF-α and inhibiting atypical immune response and release of cytokines mediated by the receptor, effectively treating AS [38].

3.6.1.2 Infliximab

Infliximab (IFX) is used to treat some diseases by boosting the immune system of the body. It is a purified, chimeric IgG monoclonal antibody protein derived from recombinant DNA that inhibits TNF-a in both murine and human components. A signaling protein called TNF-α plays a role in systemic inflammation and acute phase reactions. Neutrophils, mast cells, eosinophils, CD4+ lymphocytes, NK cells, macrophages, and neurons all produce it. By inhibiting TNF-α, the inflammatory response cascade is stopped, which improves the state of the disease (Crohn's disease, psoriasis, etc.). IFX is known to have 7–12 days of half-life in adults [39, 40]. IFX is prescribed as 5 mg/kg IV at 0, 2 and 6 weeks to AS patients. Different studies that were done to evaluate the safety and efficacy of IFX exhibited positive results. Most of the patients with the active disease when given prescribed doses of IFX showed decreased morning stiffness and acute phase reactants. Significant improvement in the QoL and bath indices (disease activity and functional ability) of the patients was observed. In addition, IFX decelerated the structural progression of the disease in AS patients [41].

Long-term treatment of AS patients with ETN has shown a reduction in the radiographic progression of the disease. Similar to IFX, treatment with ETN ensured lower levels of acute-phase reactants and improved bath indices, spinal mobility, and QoL, when compared with baseline. No adverse events (AE) or Serious AE (SAE) was observed in the patients [41].

3.6.1.3 Adalimumab

ADA is the first fully humanized recombinant IgG1 monoclonal antibody (mAb) that inhibits TNF-α to exert its effects, thereby reducing the potential for immunogenicity, in contrast to IFX, which is a chimeric antibody made up of both mouse and human domains that may trigger immune reactions that could limit its long-term use in patients with chronic conditions like rheumatoid arthritis. ADA has a very high affinity for TNF and is effective in neutralizing TNF in bioassays. The kinetic binding parameters of ADA and IFX are quite similar. Contrary ETN dissociates from TNF much more quickly [42]. ADA works by neutralizing the bioactivity of TNF-α. This is done by preventing the interaction of TNF-α with the cell surface TNF receptors. ADA is given subcutaneously in dosage of 40 mg every alternate week [43].

ADA demonstrated long-term efficacy and safety in patients with AS. ADA has exhibited greater tolerance in patients. It greatly improved the CRP levels, physical function, disease activity, and low back pain (LBP) in patients. When administered every other week, most of the patients achieved Assessment in AS response criteria (ASAS20) by week 12, and 50% of the patients achieved ASAS40 by week 52. Additionally, ADA therapy resulted in a notable reduction of acute inflammatory lesions [41].

3.6.1.4 Golimumab

Golimumab was developed by introducing human Ig genes into transgenic mice, which were then engineered to express human IgGs. Golimumab's heavy and light variable chain regions are made of an amino acid sequence that is remarkably similar to that of the human sequence (heavy chain sequence, 98%; light chain sequence, 100%). The bivalent Fab region is particular to human TNF. TNF is, therefore, less likely to circulate and bind to receptors as a result. The Fc regions' amino acid sequence matches IFX's exactly [44].

About 29 patients with active AS, a BASDAI score > 4, and a back pain score > 4 was randomized in the GO-RAISE study in a 1.8:1.8:1 ratio to receive subcutaneous injections of golimumab (50 or 100 mg) or a placebo every 4 weeks. Compared to patients in the placebo group, a significant number of patients receiving golimumab experienced an ASAS20 response (p.001) [44, 45].

Another study compared the impact of golimumab and pamidronate on MRI inflammation and clinical efficacy in AS. In a 2:1 ratio, patients who met the criteria were randomized to receive either golimumab (50 mg subcutaneously) or pamidronate (60 mg intravenously) every 4 weeks for 48 weeks. The patients also had to meet the ASAS criteria for AS and active disease (BASDAI score 4). There were recruited

30 patients. Inflammation of the spine and sacroiliac joints, as well as inflammatory markers (ESR and CRP), BASDAI, BASFI, and the Ankylosing Spondylitis Disease Activity Score (ASDAS), were significantly reduced by golimumab. Pamidronate was linked to improvements in patient-reported outcomes (PRO), and response rates to ASAS20 and ASAS40 were comparable [44–46].

3.6.1.5 Certolizumab

Certolizumab (CZP), commonly referred to as CZP pegol is a humanized antigen-binding fragment (Fab') conjugated to polyethylene glycol (PEG). It is distinct from other TNF-inhibitors because it lacks an Fc region, which reduces the possibility of Fc-mediated effects like complement-dependent cytotoxicity (CDC) or antibody-dependent cell-mediated cytotoxicity (ADCC). CZP does not induce CDC and ADCC, as shown by in vitro studies of ADA, IFX, and ETN. Additionally, in vitro research has shown that CZP inhibits lipopolysaccharide-induced cytokine production more effectively than other TNF-inhibitors, particularly ETN, and does not trigger apoptosis in activated peripheral blood lymphocytes [47].

The ASAS20 response rate at week 12 was significantly higher for the CZP 200 and 400 mg arms compared to placebo (57.7 and 63.6 vs. 38.3). A significant difference was observed at week 24 between the combined CZP arm and placebo in BASDAI (−3.05 vs. −1.05), BASFI (−2.28 vs. −0.40), and BASMI (−0.52 vs. −0.07). As early as week 1, improvements were noticed. Remarkable improvement was observed in AS subpopulation with CZP compared to placebo. Adverse events (AEs) and serious AEs were reported in 70.4 and 4.7% patients respectively in the CZP arm. No fatalities or cancers were reported [47, 48].

3.6.2 Interleukin inhibitors

Interleukins (ILs) play a significant role in the pathogenesis of AS. IL-17 has emerged to play a role in AS patients as an inflammatory mediator. Moreover, elevated serum levels of IL-17 and circulating Th17 cells have been reported in AS patients. Furthermore, endogenous interactions between IL-17A and RANKL stimulate osteoclastic activity in bone, resulting in osteoporosis, bone erosions, and osteopenia in AS patients [43, 49].

Treatment with IL-17 inhibitors (secukinumab and ixekizumab) is recommended in patients with active disease who show contraindications to TNFi. In primary non-responders to TNFi, use of IL-17 inhibitors is conditionally recommended. In patients with IBD use of IL inhibitors is not recommended. Contraindications to TNFi due to congestive heart failure or demyelinating disease, IL-17 inhibitors are preferred [20].

3.6.2.1 Secukinumab

Secukinumab is a recombinant humanized mAb that targets Interleukin-17 (IL-17), which is a proinflammatory cytokine involved in various pathological processes. Its efficacy in the management of AS has been demonstrated by many clinical trials in 2016. In addition, secukinumab has an exemplary safety profile. Secukinumab targets IL-17A specifically, thus inhibiting its binding with IL-17 receptor and cytokines expression. Therefore, normalizing the inflammation and combating pathogenic gene expression, epidermal hyper-proliferation, and T-cell infiltration. Patients with active AS who have exhibited an inadequate response to NSAIDs and TNFi therapy may benefit from secukinumab, according to the UK's National Institute for Health and Care Excellence (NICE). Secukinumab is administered under the skin, and the recommended dosage is 150 mg [50, 51].

3.6.2.2 Ixekizumab

Ixekizumab (IXE) is an IgG4 mAb, that binds to IL-17A (both IL-17A and IL-17A/F) with high specificity and affinity. IXE specifically binds to the IL-17A cytokine to block interaction with the IL17 receptor, preventing target cells from releasing proinflammatory cytokines and chemokines that have an impact on cellular components later on. IXE does not bind to the human Fc I, IIa, or IIIa receptors or to the complement subunit C1q, according to in-vitro binding tests [49].

IXE has been shown to be both safe and effective in phase II trials. In comparison to placebo-treated AS subjects, IXE-treated AS subjects had a 73% response rate for the European league against rheumatism (EULAR). Moreover, it was effective for patients who had previously failed to respond to one or more TNF inhibitors. IXE is administered subcutaneously and the recommended dosage is 160 mg every alternate week for 12 weeks, after that it can be given at a dose of 80 mg for 4 weeks [49].

3.6.3 Janus kinase inhibitors

Inflammatory and autoimmune diseases are influenced by the expression of molecules such as survival factors, chemokines, cytokines, and other molecules that promote leucocyte cell proliferation and trafficking. Since the JAK family has attracted significant interest for the potential treatment of inflammatory diseases, a variety of JAKi have been created, each with a unique selectivity profile against JAK1, JAK2, JAK3, and non-receptor tyrosine-protein kinase 2 (TYK2). The aberrant immune response is triggered by cytokines whose signal transduction is disrupted in AS [52, 53].

3.6.3.1 Tofacitinib

Tofacitinib is an orally available first-in-class pan-JAKi, which potently inhibits JAK3 and JAK1 while only weakly inhibiting JAK2 [53]. It has long been used concomitantly with MTX for the treatment of RA [54].

In a phase II trial, tofacitinib 10 mg twice daily ASAS20 response rate was predicted by the Emax model analysis of the primary endpoint to be 67.4%, 27.3% higher than the actual response rate. Tofacitinib 5 mg twice daily Assessment of Spondyloarthritis International Society 20 (ASAS 20) response rate was significantly higher than placebo (80.8 vs. 41.2%), and tofacitinib 2 and 10 mg twice daily also showed a higher response rate than placebo (51.9 and 55.8%, respectively; not significant). Secondary endpoints typically showed tofacitinib 5 and 10 mg twice daily to be more effective than placebo. The dose–response relationship was evident in objective endpoints (including MRI). There were no unexpected safety findings and adverse events were comparable between treatment groups. By week 16, dose-dependent laboratory outcome changes had nearly reached baseline [55].

Another phase III trial (NCT03502616) found that tofacitinib significantly increased the ASAS 20 response rate (56.4%) compared to placebo (29.4%) and the

ASAS 40 response rate (40.6%) compared to placebo (12.5%). Up to week 16, AEs occurred in 54.9% and 51.5% patients receiving tofacitinib and placebo, respectively. Whereby, 1.5 and 0.7% patients receiving tofacitinib and placebo respectively experienced serious AEs. When compared to a placebo, tofacitinib significantly outperformed it in treating adults with active AS. No brand-new dangers to safety were found [56].

In patients with coexisting ulcerative colitis, use of tofacitinib (approved for the treatment of ulcerative colitis) is preferred over IL-17 inhibitors if treatment with TNFi is not an option. In patients with peripheral manifestations, tofacitinib is conditionally recommended if contraindications to SSZ or MTX are exhibited [20].

3.6.3.2 Upadacitinib

It is a second-generation JAKi inhibitor that targets the JAK1 enzyme primarily. Upadacitinib works by inhibiting the Janus kinases (JAK), a family of four tyrosine kinases (JAK1, JAK2, JAK3, and TYK2) that play a role in the development of immune-mediated inflammatory diseases (IMIDs). The JAK–STAT pathway's ability to transduce growth factor- and cytokine-mediated signals intracellularly is further hampered by JAK inhibition. JAKs control gene expression, hematopoiesis, and immune cell function by phosphorylating signal transducers and activators of transcription (STATs). Upadacitinib stops STATs from becoming phosphorylated and from becoming activated inside of cells, which lessens their pro-inflammatory effects. Compared to JAK2, JAK3, and TYK2 subtypes, upadacitinib inhibits JAK1 more potently and selectively [57].

Upadacitinib 15 mg (93 patients) or a placebo (94 patients) were given to 187 patients at random. Of these, 178 (95%) patients (89 in the upadacitinib group and 89 in the placebo group) finished period 1 on the study drug. At week 14, significantly more patients in the upadacitinib group than in the placebo group had an ASAS 40 response (48%). In the upadacitinib group, 58 (62%) of 93 patients reported adverse events, compared to 52 (55%) of 94 patients in the placebo group. Creatine phosphokinase elevation was the most typical side effect in the upadacitinib group (9% of patients) (**Table 1**) [57, 59].

Cytokine therapy	Medication	FDA approval granted for treatment of AS
TNF inhibitors	Etanercept	July 2003
	Infliximab	December 2004
	Adalimumab	July 2006
	Golimumab	April 2009
	Certolizumab	October 2013
IL inhibitors	Secukinumab	January 2016
	Ixekizumab	August 2019
JAK inhibitors	Tofacitinib	December 2021
	Upadacitinib	April 2022

Table 1.
List of biologics approved by US FDA for treatment of patients with active AS [58].

4. Therapies and drug targets currently under study

4.1 Ustekinumab

The polymorphism of IL23R gene that encodes IL-23 receptor has exhibited strong association with AS, suggesting its involvement in the disease pathogenesis. Contrary to osteoarthritis patients without spinal disease, patients with active AS demonstrated higher number of IL-12, and IL-23 positive cells bone marrow of facet joints [43].

Ustekinumab is a humanized IgG1κ mAb that binds to p40-subunit commonly shared by IL-12 and IL23. It is used in the treatment of psoriatic arthritis, significantly inhibiting the radiographic progression. Since ustekinumab is well tolerated in patients, it has emerged as a novel biologic to be evaluated for the treatment of AS. In a prospective, open-label, single-arm, proof-of-concept study [treatment of patients with active AS (TOPAS)], 65% of the subjects who were administered ustekinumab achieved the primary endpoint–ASAS 40 response at week 24. Furthermore, secondary endpoints revealed clinically significant results. About 75% of the subjects achieved ASAS 20 response; in addition to 55% subjects who achieved BASDAI 50 response [53, 60].

4.2 Stem cell therapy

The first characterization of mesenchymal stem cells (MSCs) was formed in 1976. They are multipotent, meaning they have the ability to self-renew, and to differentiate into different cell types, such as adipocytes, osteoblasts, and chondrocytes. Bone marrow, umbilical cord, adipose tissue, amniotic fluid, molar cells, and peripheral blood are all sources of MSCs [61].

The efficacy and safety of MSC therapy have been demonstrated in a variety of studies, as well as in the treatment of autoimmune diseases, SLE, and MS. There are numerous clinical trials currently underway about MSC transplantation in disorders related to it, including a phase I/II clinical trial to evaluate the safety and clinical outcomes of MSC transplantation in AS patients. MSCs play important roles in immune regulation, making their transplantation a viable therapeutic option for AS patients who cannot tolerate inflammatory drug therapy. Previous studies have demonstrated that AS patients have low Treg cell counts, low B cell counts, and abnormal B cell function, with the ensuing auto-antibodies playing a role in the pathogenesis of AS [61].

5. Conclusion

NSAIDs are the first-line of treatment for patients with AS. Whereby, SSZ or other DMARDs forms the second-line treatment, and are recommended conditionally in limited clinical circumstances. In patients with no response to NSAIDs, TNF inhibitors are preferred, which tends to halt the disease progression by inhibiting the activity of TNF-α. IL inhibitors like secukinumab or ixekizumab is recommended for patients with active disease who have heart failure or demyelinating disease as a contraindication to TNF inhibitors, and in primary non-responders to TNF inhibitors. Contrary, IL inhibitors are not recommended in patients with IBD or recurrent uveitis, as TNF inhibitors are better options. Tofacitinib (JAKi) is a potential second-line option for patients with contraindications to TNF inhibitors other than infections [22]. Medications alone cannot suffice for the long term management of AS.

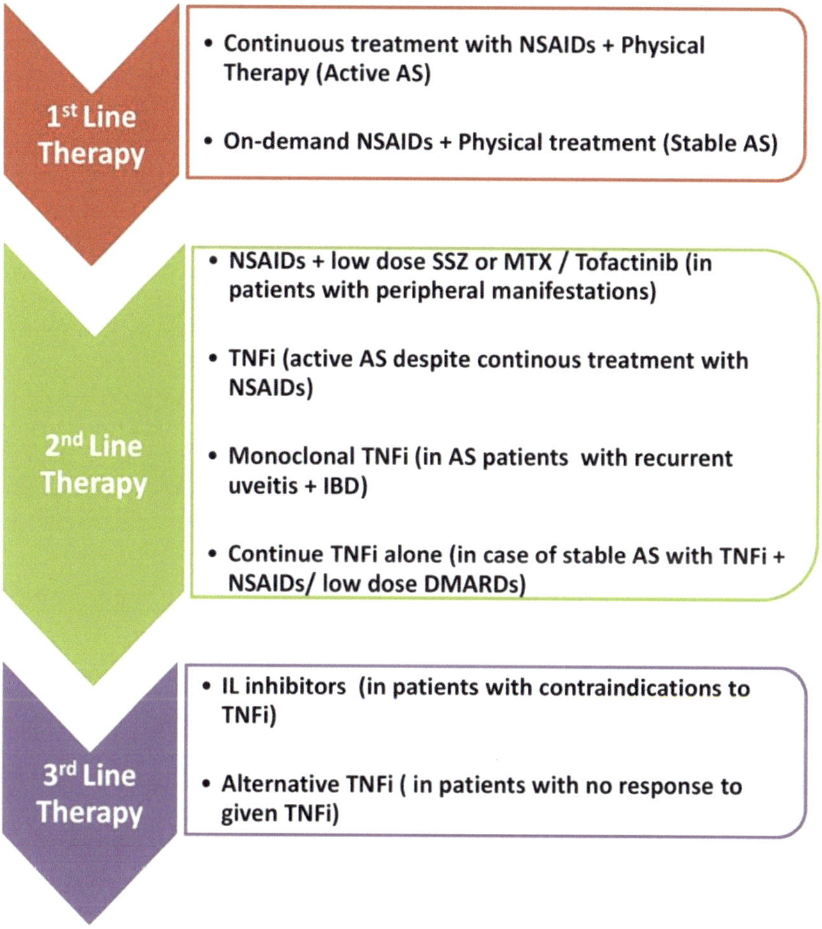

Figure 1.
Recommendations for treatment of AS given by American College of Rheumatology/Spondylitis Association of America/Spondyloarthritis Research and Treatment Network [20].

Therefore, physical therapy or yoga should be advised to the patients as it helps with improvement of AS symptoms (**Figure 1**).

Conflict of interest

The authors declare no conflict of interest.

Author details

Rajeshwar Nath Srivastava[1*], Shatakshi Pant[1], Sudeepti Ratan Srivastava[1], Amar Chandra Sharma[1] and Saloni Raj[2]

1 Department of Orthopaedic Surgery, King George's Medical University, Lucknow, UP, India

2 Westminster College, Utah, United States

*Address all correspondence to: drrnsrivastava@yahoo.com

References

[1] Mahmood F, Helliwell P. Ankylosing spondylitis: A review. EMJ. 2017;**2**(4):134-139

[2] Zhu W, He X, Cheng K, Zhang L, Chen D, Wang X, et al. Ankylosing spondylitis: Etiology, pathogenesis, and treatments. Bone Research. 2019;**7**(1). DOI: 10.1038/s41413-019-0057-8

[3] Pt CJ, PhD Pt, KS, PhD, Lmt, SJPD. Netter's Orthopaedic Clinical Examination: An Evidence-Based Approach (Netter Clinical Science). 4th ed. Elsevier; 2021

[4] Ranganathan V, Gracey E, Brown MA, Inman RD, Haroon N. Pathogenesis of ankylosing spondylitis — Recent advances and future directions. Nature Reviews Rheumatology. 2017;**13**(6):359-367. DOI: 10.1038/nrrheum.2017.56

[5] Edavalath M. Ankylosing spondylitis. Journal of Ayurveda and Integrative Medicine. Jul 2010;**1**(3):211-214. DOI: 10.4103/0975-9476.72619

[6] Golder V, Schachna L. Ankylosing spondylitis: An update. Australian Family Physician. Nov 2013;**42**(11):780-784

[7] Dean LE, Jones GT, MacDonald AG, Downham C, Sturrock RD, Macfarlane GJ. Global prevalence of ankylosing spondylitis. Rheumatology. April 2014;**53**(4):650-657. DOI: 10.1093/rheumatology/ket387

[8] News Bureau EP. Novartis, Cadila Healthcare Lead Digital Marketing Space for Ankylosing Spondylitis in India: GlobalData. Express Pharma; 2021, May 20. Available from: https://www.expresspharma.in/novartis-cadila-healthcare-lead-digital-marketing-space-for-ankylosing-spondylitis-in-india-globaldata/

[9] Zacharia B, Roy A. Ankylosing spondylitis and other seronegative arthritis. In: Connective Tissue Disease - Current State of the Art. 2020. pp. 57-68. DOI: 10.5772/intechopen.82332

[10] Gravaldi LP, Bonetti F, Lezzerini S, de Maio F. Effectiveness of physiotherapy in patients with ankylosing spondylitis: A systematic review and meta-analysis. Healthcare. 2022;**10**(1):132. DOI: 10.3390/healthcare10010132

[11] Fletcher J. Physical Therapy for Ankylosing Spondylitis: Can It Help? 2021. Available from: https://www.medicalnewstoday.com/articles/physical-therapy-for-ankylosing-spondylitis#how-can-physical-therapy-help

[12] Tricás-Moreno JM, Orosia Lucha-López M, Carmen Lucha-López A, Salavera-Bordás C, Vidal-Peracho C. Optimizing physical therapy for ankylosing spondylitis: A case study in a young football player. Journal of Physical Therapy Science. 2016;**28**(4):1392-1397. DOI: 10.1589/jpts.28.1392

[13] Aydemir K, Tok F, Peker F, Safaz I, Taskaynatan MA, Ozgul A. The effects of balneotherapy on disease activity, functional status, pulmonary function and quality of life in patients with ankylosing spondylitis. Acta Reumatológica Portuguesa. 2010 Oct-Dec;**35**(5):441-446

[14] Spondylitis Association of America. Non-Medicinal Approaches to Treating Spondyloarthritis. Spondylitis Association of America - Ankylosing Spondylitis; 2020, March 26. Available from: https://spondylitis.org/spondylitis-plus/non-medicinal-approaches-to-treating-spondyloarthritis/

[15] Singh J, Tekur P, Metri KG, Mohanty S, Singh A, Nagaratna R. Potential role of yoga in the management of ankylosing spondylitis: A retrospective study. Annals of Neurosciences. 2021;**28**(1-2):74-78. DOI: 10.1177/09727531211035335

[16] Singh J, Metri K, Tekur P, Mohanty S, Jha M, Singh A, et al. Designing, validation, and feasibility of a yoga module for patients with ankylosing spondylitis. Journal of Ayurveda and Integrative Medicine. 2022;**13**(1):100479. DOI: 10.1016/j.jaim.2021.06.019

[17] Kroon FP, van der Burg LR, Ramiro S, Landewé RB, Buchbinder R, Falzon L, et al. Non-steroidal anti-inflammatory drugs (NSAIDs) for axial spondyloarthritis (ankylosing spondylitis and non-radiographic axial spondyloarthritis). Cochrane Database of Systematic Reviews. 2015, July 17;**2015**(7). DOI: 10.1002/14651858.cd010952.pub2

[18] Taurog JD, Chhabra A, Colbert RA. Ankylosing spondylitis and axial spondyloarthritis. New England Journal of Medicine. 2016;**374**(26):2563-2574. DOI: 10.1056/nejmra1406182

[19] Toussirot E, Wendling D. Current guidelines for the drug treatment of ankylosing spondylitis. Drugs. 1998;**56**(2):225-240. DOI: 10.2165/00003495-199856020-00006

[20] Ward MM, Deodhar A, Gensler LS, Dubreuil M, Yu D, Khan MA, et al. 2019 update of the American College of Rheumatology/Spondylitis Association of America/Spondyloarthritis research and Treatment Network recommendations for the treatment of ankylosing spondylitis and nonradiographic axial spondyloarthritis. Arthritis Care & Research (Hoboken). 2019 Oct;**71**(10):1285-1299. DOI: 10.1002/acr.24025. Epub 2019 Aug 21

[21] NHS website. Treatment. Uk: Nhs; 2022, February 8. Available from: https://www.nhs.uk/conditions/ankylosing-spondylitis/treatment/

[22] Gran JT, Husby G. Ankylosing spondylitis. Drugs. 1992;**44**(4):585-603. DOI:10.2165/00003495-199244040-00006

[23] Sari S, Öztürk MA, Akkoç N. Treatment of ankylosing spondylitis. Turkish Journal of Medical Sciences. 2015;**45**:416-430. DOI: 10.3906/sag-1401-79

[24] Radu AF, Bungau SG. Management of rheumatoid arthritis: An overview. Cell. 2021;**10**(11):2857. DOI: 10.3390/cells10112857

[25] Ebrahimiadib N, Berijani S, Ghahari M, Golsoorat Pahlaviani F. Ankylosing spondylitis. Journal of Ophthalmic and Vision Research. 2021. DOI: 10.18502/jovr.v16i3.9440

[26] Chen J, Lin S, Liu C. Sulfasalazine for ankylosing spondylitis. Cochrane Database of Systematic Reviews. 2014. DOI: 10.1002/14651858.cd004800.pub3

[27] Drake MT, Clarke BL, Khosla S. Bisphosphonates: Mechanism of action and role in clinical practice. Mayo Clinic Proceedings. 2008;**83**(9):1032-1045. DOI: 10.4065/83.9.1032

[28] Toussirot R, Wendling D. Antiinflammatory treatment with bisphosphonates in ankylosing spondylitis. Current Opinion in Rheumatology. 2007;**19**(4):340-345. DOI: 10.1097/bor.0b013e328133f57b

[29] Braun J, Sieper J. Therapy of ankylosing spondylitis and other spondyloarthritides: Established medical treatment, anti-TNF-α therapy and other novel approaches. Arthritis Research. 2002;**4**(5):307. DOI: 10.1186/ar592

[30] Viapiana O, Gatti D, Idolazzi L, Fracassi E, Adami S, Troplini S, et al.

Bisphosphonates vs infliximab in ankylosing spondylitis treatment. Rheumatology. 2013;**53**(1):90-94. DOI: 10.1093/rheumatology/ket321

[31] Franks ME, Macpherson GR, Figg WD. Thalidomide. The Lancet. 2004;**363**(9423):1802-1811. DOI: 10.1016/s0140-6736(04)16308-3

[32] Ji X, Wang Y, Ma Y, Hu Z, Man S, Zhang Y, et al. Improvement of disease management and cost effectiveness in Chinese patients with ankylosing spondylitis using a smart-phone management system: A prospective cohort study. BioMed Research International. 2019;**2019**:1-11. DOI: 10.1155/2019/2171475

[33] Brandt J, Marzo-Ortega H, Emery P. Ankylosing spondylitis: New treatment modalities. Best Practice & Research. Clinical Rheumatology. 2006;**20**(3):559-570. DOI: 10.1016/j.berh.2006.03.009

[34] Braun J, van der Heijde D. Novel approaches in the treatment of ankylosing spondylitis and other spondyloarthritides. Expert Opinion on Investigational Drugs. 2003;**12**(7):1097-1109. DOI: 10.1517/13543784.12.7.1097

[35] McGregor MC, Krings JG, Nair P, Castro M. Role of biologics in asthma. American Journal of Respiratory and Critical Care Medicine. 2019;**199**(4):433-445. DOI: 10.1164/rccm.201810-1944ci

[36] Perpétuo IP, Raposeiro R, Caetano-Lopes J, Vieira-Sousa E, Campanilho-Marques R, Ponte C, et al. Effect of tumor necrosis factor inhibitor therapy on osteoclasts precursors in ankylosing spondylitis. PLoS One. 2015;**10**(12):e0144655. DOI: 10.1371/journal.pone.0144655

[37] Thomas SS, Borazan N, Barroso N, Duan L, Taroumian S, Kretzmann B, et al. Comparative immunogenicity of TNF inhibitors: Impact on clinical efficacy and tolerability in the management of autoimmune diseases. A systematic review and meta-analysis. BioDrugs. 1 August 2015;**29**(4):241-258. DOI: 10.1007/s40259-015-0134-5

[38] Wang C, Li W. Effects of etanercept and infliximab on bone metabolism indexes in patients with ankylosing spondylitis. Experimental and Therapeutic Medicine. 2019. DOI: 10.3892/etm.2019.8266

[39] Akiho H, Yokoyama A, Abe S, Nakazono Y, Murakami M, Otsuka Y, et al. Promising biological therapies for ulcerative colitis: A review of the literature. World Journal of Gastrointestinal Pathophysiology. 2015 Nov 15;**6**(4):219-227

[40] Scott FI, Lichtenstein GR. Therapeutic drug monitoring of anti-TNF therapy in inflammatory bowel disease. Current Treatment Options in Gastroenterology. 2014 Mar;**12**(1):59-75

[41] Garcia-Montoya L, Emery P. Disease modification in ankylosing spondylitis with TNF inhibitors: Spotlight on early phase clinical trials. Expert Opinion on Investigational Drugs. 2021;**30**(11):1109-1124. DOI: 10.1080/13543784.2021.2010187

[42] Salfeld J,Kupper H. Adalimumab. In: Biologics in General Medicine. 2017. pp. 14-31. DOI: 10.1007/978-3-540-29018-6_3

[43] Tahir H. Therapies in ankylosing spondylitis—From clinical trials to clinical practice. Rheumatology. 2018;**57**(Suppl_6):vi23-vi28. DOI: 10.1093/rheumatology/key152

[44] Melo AT, Campanilho-Marques R, Fonseca JE. Golimumab (anti-TNF monoclonal antibody): Where we stand today. Human Vaccines &

Immunotherapeutics. 2021 Jun 3;**17**(6):1586-1598. DOI: 10.1080/21645515.2020.1836919. Epub 2020 Dec 28

[45] Inman RD, Davis JC, van der Heijde D, Diekman L, Sieper J, Kim SI, et al. Efficacy and safety of golimumab in patients with ankylosing spondylitis: Results of a randomized, double-blind, placebo-controlled, phase III trial. Arthritis and Rheumatism. Nov 2008;**58**(11):3402-3412. DOI: 10.1002/art.23969

[46] Mok CC, Li OC, Chan KL, Ho LY, Hui PK. Effect of golimumab and pamidronate on clinical efficacy and MRI inflammation in axial spondyloarthritis: A 48-week open randomized trial. Scandinavian Journal of Rheumatology. 2015;**44**(6):480-486. DOI: 10.3109/03009742.2015.1038300

[47] Goel N, Stephens S. Certolizumab Pegol. mAbs. 2010;**2**(2):137-147. DOI: 10.4161/mabs.2.2.11271

[48] Landewé R, Braun J, Deodhar A, Dougados M, Maksymowych WP, Mease PJ, et al. Efficacy of certolizumab pegol on signs and symptoms of axial spondyloarthritis including ankylosing spondylitis: 24-week results of a double-blind randomised placebo-controlled phase 3 study. Annals of the Rheumatic Diseases. Jan 2014;**73**(1):39-47. DOI: 10.1136/annrheumdis-2013-204231. Epub 2013 Sep 6

[49] Benucci M, Damiani A, Li Gobbi F, Grossi V, Infantino M, Manfredi M, et al. Therapeutic potential of Ixekizumab in the treatment of ankylosing spondylitis: A review on the emerging clinical data. Therapeutics and Clinical Risk Management. 2020;**16**:287-297. DOI: 10.2147/tcrm.s228880

[50] Aboobacker S, Kurn H, Al Aboud AM. Secukinumab. In: StatPearls [Internet]. Treasure Island (FL): StatPearls Publishing; 2022 Apr 30

[51] Blair HA. Secukinumab: A review in ankylosing spondylitis. Drugs. 2019;**79**(4):433-443. DOI: 10.1007/s40265-019-01075-3

[52] Thompson C, Davies R, Choy E. Anti cytokine therapy in chronic inflammatory arthritis. Cytokine. 2016;**86**:92-99. DOI: 10.1016/j.cyto.2016.07.015

[53] XELJANZ. Summary of Product Characteristics. Pfizer Ltd

[54] National Center for Biotechnology Information. Pub Chem Compound Summary for CID 9926791, Tofacitinib. 2022. Retrieved July 12, 2022 from https://pubchem.ncbi.nlm.nih.gov/compound/Tofacitinib

[55] van der Heijde D, Deodhar A, Wei JC, Drescher E, Fleishaker D, Hendrikx T, et al. Tofacitinib in patients with ankylosing spondylitis: A phase II, 16-week, randomised, placebo-controlled, dose-ranging study. Annals of the Rheumatic Diseases. 2017 Aug;**76**(8):1340-1347. DOI: 10.1136/annrheumdis-2016-210322. Epub 2017 Jan 27

[56] Deodhar A, Sliwinska-Stanczyk P, Xu H, Baraliakos X, Gensler LS, Fleishaker D, et al. Tofacitinib for the treatment of ankylosing spondylitis: A phase III, randomised, double-blind, placebo-controlled study. Annals of the Rheumatic Diseases. 2021;**80**(8):1004-1013. DOI: 10.1136/annrheumdis-2020-219601

[57] Padda IS, Bhatt R, Parmar M. Upadacitinib. [updated 2022 Jan 6]. In: StatPearls [Internet]. Treasure Island (FL): StatPearls Publishing; Jan 2022

[58] CenterWatch. Ankylosing Spondylitis | FDA Approved Drugs | CenterWatch. n.d. Available from: https://www.Centerwatch.Com/Directories/1067-Fda-Approved-Drugs/Topic/550-Ankylosing-Spondylitis

[59] van der Heijde D, Song IH, Pangan AL, Deodhar A, van den Bosch F, Maksymowych WP, et al. Efficacy and safety of upadacitinib in patients with active ankylosing spondylitis (SELECT-AXIS 1): A multicentre, randomised, double-blind, placebo-controlled, phase 2/3 trial. Lancet. 7 Dec 2019;**394**(10214):2108-2117. DOI: 10.1016/S0140-6736(19)32534-6. Epub 2019 Nov 12

[60] Poddubnyy D, Hermann K-GA, Callhoff J, Listing J, Sieper J. Ustekinumab for the treatment of patients with active ankylosing spondylitis: Results of a 28-week, prospective, open-label, proof-of-concept study (TOPAS). Annals of the Rheumatic Diseases. 2014;**73**:817-823

[61] Abdolmohammadi K, Pakdel FD, Aghaei H, Assadiasl S, Fatahi Y, Rouzbahani NH, et al. Ankylosing spondylitis and mesenchymal stromal/stem cell therapy: A new therapeutic approach. Biomedicine & Pharmacotherapy. 2019;**109**:1196-1205. DOI: 10.1016/j.biopha.2018.10.137